ADVANCE PRAISE FOR
BANISHING NIGHT TERRORS AND NIGHTMARES

"A unique and significant contribution to an in-depth understanding of the perplexing world of night terrors. Absolute must reading for professionals in the field as well as for victims and their families."

—Caroll Yap, M.D., Staff Psychiatrist, California Department of Corrections; previously Assistant Clinical Professor of Medicine, University of California–Irvine; psychiatrist, Cambridge University, Cambridge, England; psychotherapist, Boarding School for Maladjusted Children, Cambridge, England

BANISHING NIGHT TERRORS AND NIGHTMARES

A BREAKTHROUGH PROGRAM TO HEAL THE TRAUMAS THAT SHATTER PEACEFUL SLEEP

Christopher Raoul Carranza
and
Jane R. Dill, Ph.D., L.M.F.T., D.A.P.A.

KENSINGTON BOOKS
www.kensingtonbooks.com

KENSINGTON BOOKS are published by

Kensington Publishing Corp.
850 Third Avenue
New York, NY 10022

Permission to use the following material is gratefully acknowledged:
From *High Risk: Children Without a Conscience* by Carole McKelvey and Kevin Magid, copyright © 1987 by Dr. Kevin Magid and Carole A. McKelvey. Used by permission of Bantam Books, a division of Random House, Inc.

From *Dreams and Nightmares: The Origin and Meaning of Dreams* by Ernest Hartmann, M.D., copyright © 1998 by Ernest Hartmann, published by Perseus Book Group. Used by permission.

From *Rebuilding Shattered Lives* by James A. Chu, M.D., copyright © 1998 by James A. Chu. This material is used by permission of John Wiley & Sons, Inc.

All Kensington titles, imprints, and distributed lines are available at special quantity discounts for bulk purchases for sales promotions, premiums, fund-raising, educational, or institutional use.

Special book excerpts or customized printings can also be created to fit specific needs. For details, write or phone the office of the Kensington special sales manager: Kensington Publishing Corp., 850 Third Avenue, New York, NY 10022, attn: Special Sales Department; phone: 1-800-221-2647.

Kensington and the K logo are Reg. U.S. Pat. & TM Off.

ISBN 0-7582-0542-2

First printing: March 2004

10 9 8 7 6 5 4 3 2 1

Printed in the United States of America

With special thanks to
Charles Edward Carranza, M.A.
in appreciation for his
invaluable assistance
throughout the writing of this book

Contents

Preface

This book has come about as the result of a long and difficult journey. From late in my first year of life until over four decades later I suffered from severe ongoing night terrors. In my thirties, after much unsuccessful professional intervention, my desperation and frustration drove me to try a different approach in order to make some sense out of this lifelong horror show that had been devastating my sleep and my life for all those years. I began a long-term program of intensive research, documentation, and investigation. Some ten years later, the resulting plethora of information I had assembled yielded solutions that led to the cessation of my night terror problem.

In an effort to share what I had learned in the process, I began organizing my night terror research and writings into articles and finally into a book. After working on all of those for several years, I came to realize that something was missing. While they comprehensively addressed long-term trauma and night terrors, they did not adequately cover the related subjects of short-term trauma and repetitive nightmares. I felt that Dr. Jane Dill, a professional I had known for several years, would be an excellent choice to fill in what was missing. In addition to other projects, we had already collaborated on an article about sleep disorders that was published by the American Association for Marriage and Family Therapy in 1999.

We soon decided that we could make the greatest positive impact by co-authoring the final version of this book. Chapters 1 through 13 are based upon my own experiences, research, and solutions, with primary emphasis upon all types of night terrors in both children and adults, while Dr. Dill's chapters 14 through 16 are based upon her extensive background as a professional therapist, with specific focus upon the current outbreak of nightmares and other sleep disorders arising from short-term, single-incident trauma such as the terrorist attacks of 9/11. This makes our book the first to deal comprehensively with the many connecting threads, understandings, and workable strategies for combating the insidious and perplexing maladies addressed herein.

We wrote this book for a wide variety of interested readers— night terror and nightmare sufferers and those close to them, medical professionals, therapists, psychologists, and psychiatrists. However, even if a reader's interest is primarily motivated by a desire to find solutions to the many problems created by recent traumatic events such as 9/11, it is essential, in order to fully comprehend and effectively treat any type of trauma-related sleep disorder, to become thoroughly familiar with the entire book.

Throughout these pages there are different levels of depth, emphasis, and direction. By carefully reading it, the layman, the nightmare or night terror sufferer, and the professional will come to recognize the immediate as well as the long-term ramifications associated with these disorders. They will also discover that workable solutions actually exist, even for the most severe and persistent of long-term night terrors, which have commonly been thought to be incurable. The book clearly illuminates the existence of far too much misinformation and too many incomplete, erroneous, and ill-informed points of view. As famed sleep disorder specialist Dr. William Dement (1999) wrote: "My most significant finding is that ignorance is the worst sleep disorder of them all." (1, p.9)*

Almost all nightmare and night terror victims and their families experience years of suffering and frustration, from the condition that is tearing their lives apart and from the lack of any truly helpful information and/or solutions. While the suffering may seem unavoidable at present, the frustration is completely unnecessary! There already exists an exhaustive, largely overlooked fifty-year wealth of accurate published information on these subjects. Bringing this virtual flood of ignored information to the attention of sufferers and professionals alike has been one of our primary purposes in writing this book. Therefore, many relevant portions of the valuable existing information buried in the professional archives will be quoted, explored, and explained.

While we are confident that our book is the most helpful and informative source currently available on the subject of night terrors, as well as a great aid to those who suffer from repetitive nightmares, we do not pretend to be the final authorities. Our position is similar to that of Dr. M. Scott Peck (1983), who wrote at the beginning of *People of the Lie,* "Do not regard anything written here as the last word. Indeed, the purpose of the book is to lead us to dissatisfaction with our current state of ignorance on the subject." (2, p.10)

Christopher R. Carranza
Garden Grove, California

*Numbered references refer to the list on pages 223–28.

Acknowledgments

Dr. Dill would like to thank the following people for their valuable input: Ralph Downey III, Ph.D., director, and Wesley Elon Fleming, M.D., of the Loma Linda University Sleep Disorder Center, and also Wilma Bradley, B.S.N., Penny Watkins, B.S.N., and Elaine Weiner, M.S.

A SUFFERER'S JOURNEY

by Christopher Raoul Carranza

Part One

Chapter 1

The Two Distinct Types of Night Terrors

The prestigious *Diagnostic and Statistical Manual of Mental Disorders* (*DSM* IV) makes a clear distinction between those childhood night terror disorders which are not the result of psychopathology and thus resolve themselves spontaneously, and the night terror disorders which either continue into, or even begin in adulthood. The adult condition is stated to be a result of serious psychopathology and therefore does not resolve itself.

The DSM IV says: "Children with [Night] Terror Disorder do not have a higher incidence of psychopathology or mental disorders than does the general population. Psychopathology is more likely to be associated with [Night] Terror Disorder in adults . . . [Night] Terror Disorder begins in children between ages 4 and 12 years and resolves spontaneously during adolescence. In adults, it most commonly begins between ages 20 and 30 years and often follows a chronic course, with the frequency and severity of episodes waxing and waning over time." (3, pp.585, 586)*

All the studies proving that extreme child abuse results in consistent biological changes, which lead to later anxiety disorders, are only relevant to severe-trauma-related night terrors and have nothing to do with the night terror condition exclusive to child-

*See the numbered list of references, page 223–28.

hood. This discovery has given me a basis for accurately labeling these two quite distinct conditions for the first time. The temporary condition that is relatively common in childhood and ultimately resolves itself will be called "Type A Night Terrors," while the rarer, extreme-trauma-related condition (which may begin either in childhood or adulthood) that has routinely resisted treatment for the entire lifetime of the individual will be called "Type B Night Terrors." This essential update in terminology will make the explanations in this book much easier to follow.

Previously, even those researchers who recognized that these were two different conditions had to express themselves through unclear, confusing terminology. If I were to adhere to the current inconsistent terminology throughout this book, then a juvenile experiencing trauma-related adult night terrors would be referred to by the misleading oxymoron, "a child adult night terror sufferer." But it can now be clearly stated that *the great majority of childhood night terror victims are suffering from Type A Night Terrors that will go away by themselves. Only that small minority of children who experience extreme brutal abuse in infancy and/or childhood and have their brain chemistry altered are suffering from the trauma-related Type B Night Terrors that will persist for the lifetime of the individual, if left untreated.*

Nothing has caused more confusion than the incorrect labeling of Type A Night Terrors and Type B Night Terrors as the same condition. The symptoms may look the same when experienced by children, but they are not indicative of the same condition. Those who are watching their own children being thrashed about by night terrors are usually quite frantic. It is a very difficult thing to watch. The good news is that if you are highly upset by watching your child suffer from this malady, then the problem is most likely the nonserious, casually caused, shallow rooted, self-resolving Type A Night Terror condition. This is in sharp contrast to the serious, usually maliciously caused, deeply rooted, extremely resistant, and much rarer Type B Night Terror problem.

Everything about Type B Night Terrors is so far removed from the conventional spectrum of human experience that in order to intimately know this enigmatic malady, one would almost certainly have to be living with it or have lived with it. My own foundation and understandings stem from having suffered from the condition for over forty years and having extensively documented and studied the two types of night terrors for approximately fifteen of those years. All of this experience and research was required in order to arrive at the solutions which have allowed me finally to be free of Type B Night Terrors for the first time in my life.

Although astute researchers had been writing about the link between extreme trauma and Type B Night Terrors for over fifty years, their peers failed to take the time to follow their chain of deductive reasoning and logic in order to verify these experts' contentions. I was fortunate that it was on my watch that science finally caught up with truth.

The first definitive study on the relationship between extreme child abuse and the later development of adult anxiety disorders was published just after the first draft of this book had been completed. The August 2, 2000, issue of *The Journal of the American Medical Association (JAMA)* contained the article "Pituitary-Adrenal and Autonomic Responses to Stress in Women After Sexual and Physical Abuse in Childhood." Advanced diagnostic procedures showed that extreme child abuse consistently results in chemical changes to the child's brain. More important, the brain damage sustained in childhood was found to play a role in the later development of a number of disorders in adulthood. Among these are "mood and anxiety disorders . . . panic disorder . . . PTSD . . . depression" and "disruption of sleep." (4, pp.592, 593)

The findings discussed above, as well as other recent information, are necessary in order to begin effectively diagnosing and treating sleep disorders. In a disturbing study, Dr. William Dement found that "Somewhere between 95 and 99 percent of all sleep disorder sufferers in 1991, and today in 1998, remain undiagnosed and untreated or misdiagnosed and mistreated. That is millions and millions of people." (1, p.354) He also wrote: "Generally, these cases are handled by psychiatrists. Although . . .

most of them have no expertise in sleep disorders." (1, p.144) Their lack of expertise in regard to night terrors has led psychiatrists to assume that all childhood night terror victims are suffering from the nonserious, shallow rooted, nonpsychologically aberrant, self-resolving Type A condition. This oversight has been highly detrimental to the children who were actually suffering from trauma-related Type B Night Terrors. Only after the malady has persisted into adulthood does the patient's night terror problem reveal itself to be serious, deeply rooted, psychologically aberrant, and highly resistant to treatment, and by then the opportunity for early intervention has passed.

Sleep disorders in general are a relatively recent, narrow, oftentimes nebulous area of study, and night terrors in particular are a microcosm within that already limited field. Therefore, it is not surprising that much of the existing night terror literature is conflicting and confusing. The pervasive darkness that has always surrounded this obscure subject can only be breached through open-minded humility, a willingness to question the status quo, and an honest admission that current understandings are less than conclusive. Dr. Dement accurately stated: "The current way, or non-way [in which we deal with sleep disorders] is so very bad." He also wrote: "For nearly half a century, a huge reservoir of knowledge about sleep disorders has been building up behind a dam of pervasive lack of awareness and unresponsive bureaucracies. It is time to blow up the dam." (1, pp.4, 10, 144)

Although Dr. Dement is referring to all sleep disorders, with night terrors per se, this demolition process has to begin with the widespread recognition that Type A Night Terrors and Type B Night Terrors are not the same condition. This unfortunate misunderstanding has consistently undermined the literary continuity and theoretical consistency of all but a few writings on the subject. How can the same condition be simultaneously a nonserious childhood idiosyncrasy and also an extremely serious lifelong malady? How is it possible that the same disease is reported to resolve itself by the time the sufferer reaches adolescence and at the same time is found to resist decades of the most advanced professional intervention? How can the same disorder simultaneously have unknown origins thought to be rooted in genetics, while also having its origins recently documented and conclusively found to be rooted in extreme environmental trauma? How can the same malady be a shallow rooted, transient developmental phase unrelated to any psychopathological condition and at the same time be a deeply rooted, neurobiological aberration just now discovered to include measurable brain damage at the chemical level?

Is it possible for a single condition to evidence all these contradictory characteristics? Certainly not. Therefore, once that is recognized, then the inconsistencies dissipate. Type A Night Terrors are a temporary idiosyncrasy that is not uncommon among children. The condition has no documented origins, is not indicative of serious psychopathology, is shallow rooted, and will usually resolve itself before adolescence without any professional intervention whatsoever. On the other hand, Type B Night Terrors are a much rarer, lifelong malady now proven to be a persistent consequence of extreme trauma. The condition is deeply rooted and is indicative of serious psychopathology. Therefore, Type B Night Terrors will not abate by themselves. And the discovery of documented brain damage explains why decades of professional intervention have failed to combat this condition.

The designations "childhood night terrors" and "adult night terrors" speak more about the age of the sufferer than they do about the characteristics of the malady. Since children can also suffer from the trauma-related condition, both terms are inaccurate and misleading. Therefore, there is nothing revolutionary about correctly labeling these two diverse conditions; the professional literature has been drawing this distinction for decades. Back in 1987, few people listened when Susan Knapp wrote: "The second type 2 night terrors are called the traumatic type because they begin in response to acute physical or emotional trauma. They can occur in a *child* of any age and are quite similar to dreams of adults who are suffering from traumatic war neurosis." She also voiced a profound truth when writing: "It is not surprising that attitudes of parents versus professionals toward the incidence of night terrors in children differ considerably. Many professionals see this disorder as a temporary childhood idiosyncrasy, which they feel the child will outgrow. Moreover, almost all writers consider that night terrors in adults are quite serious." (5, p.183)

Dr. Dement concurred with Knapp when he wrote: "About three percent of children experience night terrors, although many cases are probably not tabulated. Night terrors occur most often in children between two and five years of age and usually disappear completely by age seven. The disorder also may appear late in life, probably due to a form of epilepsy or organic changes in the brain." (1, p.213) Lydia Dotto added: "[Night terrors] are usually outgrown by adolescence. If they occur in adults, they are considered more serious because they may be symptomatic of psychological problems." (6, p.117) Wilise Webb also agreed with the above cited writers when stating: "While [night terrors] are likely to be terrifying to concerned parents, they appear to be a momentary and apparently unconscious part of the child's concern . . . best viewed as part of growing up. Night terrors in rare instances may persist or emerge in adults at disturbing levels. The findings in these cases indicate that these episodes typically involve psychological problems and therapeutic help is needed." (7, p.100)

Clearly, the professional literature has repeatedly drawn a distinction between non-serious Type A (true childhood) Night Terrors and serious Type B (trauma-related) Night Terrors. It appears that even legal systems around the world have been aware of the difference. Wilise Webb wrote: "A British man was acquitted of murder after strangling his wife while in the throes of a night terror involving defending himself against attack by two Japanese soldiers." (7, p.118) Would the British courts have been so lenient had they viewed this man's condition as some temporary idiosyncrasy, phase, or quirk?

Others have noted some of the same discrepancies indicated above. Dr. John Marshall wrote: "It is not clear whether night terrors in children are the same phenomenon as they are in adults, although they appear quite similar clinically." (8, p.294) The three adult patients Dr. Marshall documents in his study developed night terrors after exposure to extreme trauma. The first patient developed night terrors after life-threatening complications following surgery. The second experienced a construction-related electrocution accident that threw him from atop a building and broke his back. The third suffered trauma to the head from a severe industrial accident. (8, pp.293, 294) All three documented cases are definitely examples of Type B Night Terrors.

Dr. Marshall knew the origins of the Type B Night Terrors in all three of his patients. He documented the clear link between extreme trauma and the onset of this type of night terrors. He was aware of the fact that Type A Night Terrors have no clear link with extreme trauma. That is probably why he questioned whether the childhood condition was the same phenomenon in spite of similar appearances.

Just as plentiful as the literature stating that Type A Night Terrors go away by themselves is the literature stating that Type B Night Terrors are relatively resistant to treatment. Over fifty years after the last concentration camp was liberated, and after years of psychotherapy, Holocaust survivors are still suffering from Type B Night Terrors. The entire medical community has had trouble curing Type B Night Terror sufferers whether the root trauma was the result of child abuse, the Holocaust, a POW camp, a war situation, torture, or a marine or other life-threatening accident or scenario. Presently, we have an additional source of Type B Night Terrors developing as a result of the terrorist atrocities that occurred in America on 9/11/01.

The writings of Eitinger and Schwarz are an accurate description of the Type B Night Terror treatment failures of the world-wide psychiatric/psychological community. They wrote: "We know today that the problem has not diminished . . . since then [WW II]. Reports from all over the world indicate that traditional psychotherapy (including Freudian psychoanalysis) is insufficient." (9, p.218) The studies of abused children, Holocaust survivors, prisoners of war, World War II and Korean war veterans, shipwrecked mariners, Vietnam veterans, victims of severe accidents, as well as of many other scenarios are not sporadic or isolated cases. They represent thousands of individuals in which various forms of extreme psychic trauma resulted in the development of Type B Night Terrors, which persisted and still persist for the lifetime of the individual.

While Type A Night Terrors go away by themselves, the best that has been achieved for Type B sufferers is a masking of the symptoms with drugs. As Wilise Webb wrote: "No amount of [drugs] will cure the troubled mind. Unless time, circumstances, or our own efforts have removed the pressures which require the use of the drug, those pressures will continue; they have been only temporarily masked." (7, pp.126, 127) Those pressures will not be relieved until the treating practitioners begin to understand the staggering depth of the problem.

The true traumatic origins, extreme depth, and lifelong ramifications of Type B Night Terrors are only now starting to be recognized and documented. Some of these crucial factors were revealed in 1997 when Dr. Carol Glod released a groundbreaking study on sleep disturbances in severely abused children. She wrote: "Child abuse has been associated with a variety of psychiatric sequelae, including post traumatic stress disorder (PTSD). The hallmarks of the state include re-experience of the trauma. . . . Sleep is often affected by recurring distressing dreams as part of the re-experience phenomenon. . . . Childhood physical abuse is a common traumatic experience, often presumed to be associated with sleep disruption and nightmares." (10, p.1236)

Recently there has been a virtual flood of data on these issues. Unfortunately, this information has been dispersed throughout the medical, sociological, psychological, psychiatric, pediatric, and child abuse journals, in addition to conventional mainstream periodicals. Too often professionals begin practice and either stop reading or have too little time to keep up with the literature in their own field, much less the literature of other fields. So psychiatrists treating Type B Night Terror victims may not even be aware of the cutting-edge literatures. As a result, some remain reluctant to let go of past misconceptions about the diagnosis and treatment of the malady, or even to investigate the proven findings which discredit these mistaken and outdated ideas.

Another reason that misunderstandings about all night terrors have flourished is that much of the early literature and even some of the later studies use the terms nightmare and night terror interchangeably. Kales and associates wrote: "Night terrors have often been confused with nightmares, and the variations in use of these two terms in the literature have added to this confusion." (13, p.1413) Even in the same article, the terms are sometimes used interchangeably. In 1973 Fisher and associates wrote: "Of 200 volunteers, only those with an alleged frequency of three or more nightmares per week were chosen for study. None of the night terror subjects selected were overly psychotic." (14, p.77) Fisher and associates were clearly referring to night terrors in this entire quote. Similarly, although often using the term nightmares, Eitinger was distinctly describing the symptoms of trauma-related Type B Night Terrors in all of his concentration camp writings.

Regrettably, most of those currently attempting to treat night terror victims are unable to distinguish the symptoms or determine the causes essential to correctly diagnose whether the patient is suffering from Type A Night Terrors, Type B Night Terrors, or nightmares. These symptoms and causes will be thoroughly explored in later chapters.

Nightmares will be addressed in Dr. Dill's section of this book. However, generally, in contrast to night terrors, nightmares have the following characteristics: They (1) occur naturally; (2) are mostly cerebral events that take place in REM sleep and can occur at any time of night (night terrors occur in the deepest stages of non-REM sleep, and the most intense attacks are almost always within the first hour of sleep); (3) are marked by a protective paralysis over the body that limits the physical intensity and outward actions of the sleeper—sufferers are usually incapable of seriously injuring or killing themselves or others (night terror sufferers have done both); (4) occur in children and adults; (5) have onset in childhood or adulthood, and (6) this onset may follow an actual con-corn or a traumatizing experience, or may be in response to something as benign as a scary story or movie; (7) are usually intermittent, but in rarer cases may recur over months or years; (8) are universally common—virtually everyone has had a nightmare; (9) unless recurring, as a result of a traumatizing experience, require no treatment; even when recurring, can be dealt with directly because nightmares take place in a lower level of unconsciousness than night terrors—unlike night terrors, the content and theme of the nightmare can be clearly remembered; (10) they have a variety of causes; and there are (11) generally, no altered brain chemistry; (12) generally, no indication of psychopathology; (13) no consistent related personality traits; (14) no serious related health problems; (15) generally, no related interpersonal problems; and (16) relatively normal emotional range.

The following chart summarizes the salient characteristics of Type A and Type B Night Terrors as discussed throughout this book:

Type A Night Terrors	Type B Night Terrors
1. Not genetically caused	1. Not genetically caused
2. Unique pattern of extreme attacks	2. Unique pattern of extreme attacks
3. Far more intense than nightmares	3. Far more intense than nightmares
4. Exclusive to children	4. Occurs in children and adults
5. Onset only in childhood	5. Onset in childhood or adulthood
6. Onset follows mundane experience	6. Onset follows extreme trauma
7. Temporary even if not treated	7. Virtually permanent if not treated
8. Relatively common	8. Less common
9. Self-resolving	9. Must be effectively treated
10. Either nontraumatic causes or relatively short-lived or low-level traumas that are magnified by the sufferer's limited emotional development	10. Extremely traumatic causes
11. No altered brain chemistry	11. Definite altered brain chemistry
12. Not indicative of psychopathology	12. Indicative of psychopathology
13. No consistent personality traits	13. Consistent personality traits
14. No other related health problems	14. Serious related health problems
15. No related interpersonal problems	15. Definite interpersonal problems
16. Relatively normal emotional range	16. Extremely repressed emotions

Chapter 2

A Unique Story

Although Type B Night Terrors have been a part of my life as far back as I can remember, I did not begin my life with that condition. From the hospital in which I was born, I was taken directly to a well-run Catholic orphanage and lovingly cared for by a woman named Rose Carino.

I had been placed in the orphanage by my biological parents. My mother (Gladys) had been four months pregnant with me when she married my father (Raoul). From the wedding day until my birth, Gladys avoided all contact with family and friends so that no one would see that she was pregnant.

Shortly after my birth, I was hastily named Raoul (the same name as my father) and whisked away to the orphanage. My parents could return home, resume contact with family and friends (after being in seclusion for five months), and "wash their hands" of the events of the previous year.

Gladys almost immediately became pregnant with my sister Geraldine. I was born in December of 1953; Geraldine was to be born in October of 1954. Guilt, conscience, or some other motive caused Raoul to threaten Gladys with a poorly conceived ultimatum. He told her privately that if she did not agree to adopt me from the orphanage, he would end the marriage, leave her three months pregnant with Geraldine, and tell her family and friends the whole truth.

This volatile woman, who herself had suffered an extremely abusive childhood at the hands of an alcoholic father, was now being blackmailed into accepting the job of mother to an un-wanted five-month-old infant whom she had assumed she would never have to deal with again. It would have been out of the ques-tion for her to allow her husband to go through with his threats. Therefore, she was forced to accept being chained to the oars of motherhood at a time when she was even more volatile than usual.

Then, in order to cover up their previous subterfuge, Gladys and Raoul decided to lie again to friends and family by telling them that they were adopting a total stranger. Since they had had no intention of taking me back when they originally handed me over for adoption, the hasty choice of the name Raoul hadn't mattered at the time. However, now there was a problem caused by my having been given that particular name. The fact that this alleged "complete stranger" already had the same rare ethnic name as the new adopting father was too transparent a coincidence! So, they decided to solve that problem by renaming me Christopher. They would later make this name legal, just before I entered kinder-garten.

For the first five months of my life, I had been in the care of a compassionate, loving Catholic orphanage worker who met my needs, gave me love, and called me Raoul. Correspondingly, the orphanage records indicate a normal baby, happy and healthy, with no indication of sleep disturbances or any other abnormali-ties.

After five months, I woke up one morning in a strange home with an angry, hostile woman who called me Christopher instead of Raoul. My father, who had insisted on bringing me back from the orphanage, was not around to protect me because he had his own life, including other women outside of the home. This fur-ther infuriated Gladys, who had no one around upon whom to vent her frustrations except me. She was stuck in a miserable, hellish situation for which she took no responsibility. In her own mind, she truly believed that she was the victim and that I was to blame for this entire mess. She saw the pregnancy that began this dismal chain of events as my fault, not hers. I subsequently became the target of her almost constant torturous psychopathic rampages.

While it's virtually impossible to accurately describe my own interaction with this incredibly sadistic woman, especially in regard to the earliest years, her continuous actions toward the other four people in the household (three planned children and her husband) tell a little about Gladys's capacity for malevolence. Two knife-and-milk-bottle-throwing incidents stand out, along with the time she slowly lowered her youngest child's hand onto a hot stove in order to extract a confession for a minor offense. Raging, screaming, punching, kicking, and cursing for hours were part of the ongoing daily routine for more than a decade. Bloody marathon beatings with bats and other objects were commonplace. Squirting her husband and the couch where he slept with lighter fluid and threatening to set him ablaze, as well as threatening to scald him with boiling water: These were typical of the many scenes that took place intermittently for years.

But these examples fall short of conveying to the reader a true feeling for the continual consummate hatred this woman reserved exclusively for me when no one else was around. In a relative sense, and compared to the far more hostile actions she perpetrated against me in private, the behaviors described above constitute her controlled, audience-conscious anger. I'm quite convinced that this brutal environment was the root cause of my long-term Type B Night Terror problem.

The normal love, bonding, and attachment to Rose Carino at the orphanage were among the greatest blessings of my life. Without the attachment that preceded the extreme child abuse, I might have been on track to develop into an angry psychopath and abusive parent myself. Gladys was raised in an abusive, dysfunctional home. There is currently a great deal of evidence to suggest that infants who do not initially experience love, bonding, and attachment grow up to be the permanently detached, angry, conscienceless, empty, and often dangerous adults of tomorrow. Almost all of the Ted Bundys and Charles Mansons of the world experienced horrendous abuse early on in life and lacked even the short period of bonding that I experienced at the orphanage. However, this bonding cannot prevent extreme trauma from causing dire consequences in terms of later anxiety disorders.

Type B Night Terrors and extreme brutal abuse were my constant companions during childhood. During early adolescence, my rapid increase in height and strength put an end to the extreme physical abuse I had experienced for all those years, but the night terrors continued. Neither of my parents sought any help for my condition. This was certainly because they feared exposure of the heinous things that were going on inside the home.

Although my Type B Night Terrors continued well into adulthood, I was surprisingly successful and functional in every area of my life—except relationships and emotional issues. This is typical of Type B sufferers and will be discussed at greater length later on in this book.

Finally, in my thirties, the lack of sleep and extreme disruption of my life caused me to seek professional help for my night terror problem, but this only caused the problem to become worse. The frustration of trying to find consistent accurate information as well as competent professional help was also turning my waking hours into a nightmare. Rather than expertise, the multitude of professionals from whom I sought help and information did not even possess a minimal understanding of night terrors. One doctor in particular was especially inept and yet had been "treating" night terror victims for years. His shortcomings went undetected by his patients largely because individuals who must turn to the mental health profession for help are often the very people least able to make cognizant judgments about the competency and sincerity of those they've entrusted with their lives.

But everyone, even the more conscientious professionals, dismissed my background as completely unrelated to the problem. "Night terrors are genetic," I was told. "Outside of that, we know very little." Having experienced night terrors for these many decades, I couldn't help but see a link between the extreme, otherworldly emotional intensity of an actual night terror attack and the extreme emotional and physical trauma that I suffered during childhood. Since the professionals with whom I was dealing had never personally experienced a night terror attack, they knew nothing about how truly intense an episode can be. Therefore, it was easy for them to adhere to prevailing theory and not make a connection between my past and my present. They were the experts, so I accepted their assessments. However, several years of sleep labs, psychotherapy, other counseling, hypnosis, etc., yielded no positive results. This was because, after the condition was diagnosed, no one seemed to have any truly effective answers.

Since the professionals I encountered were almost as much in the dark as I was, I decided to start keeping several detailed and extensive logs. Although I did not realistically expect any substantial results from this procedure, I needed at least to feel that I was trying to do something for myself. I also contacted the Catholic orphanage in which I had spent my first five months of life. To my surprise, Rose Carino was still there. Speaking to this kind and loving woman was tremendously informative and heartwarming. But something about our conversation was noticeably unusual. After almost thirty-five years, Rose Carino remembered every single detail of this case as if it had happened yesterday. She described the two parents I was placed with as if they were standing right in front of her. Everything about the physical appearance, mannerisms, and circumstances of these two insincere, disturbed people was permanently etched into her mind.

One of the logs I had started eventually contained everything I could remember about my childhood and past, including the information obtained from Rose. Another contained everything about my daily activities. I noted information about work, exercise, interpersonal dealings, sex, diet, caffeine, and almost everything that happened during the day. In yet another log I recorded everything about the night: what time I went to bed, what time I woke up, hours of sleep, quality of sleep, and most important, details about the night terror attack, if one had occurred that night. Since I was experiencing an average of four to six night terrors per week, and there were evenings of multiple episodes, this log contained a great deal of information. I was looking for any kind of link between my daily activities and the occurrence of a terror attack that night.

After several years of this, all I seemed to have were thousands of pieces of paper. That's when the most helpful log of all began to pay dividends. This log showed that my own experience paralleled certain outstanding accounts to be found in the professional literature. I had been collecting all the literature I could find on night terrors, as well as on post-traumatic stress disorder (PTSD). One group of diverse articles carried a consistent theme. Several of the articles about Holocaust survivors, one about the survivors of a marine disaster, one about some Vietnam veterans, and several others about the victims of the Chowchilla, California, kidnapping—all attributed the development of night terrors to the victims' having experienced severe psychic trauma.

I had finally pinpointed the literature that convincingly validated my own certainty about the relationship between my torturous childhood and a lifetime of night terrors. From there, I contacted a sleep disorder expert I had seen on the Oprah Winfrey show on April 6, 1996. He told me about a drug called Klonopin which is sometimes effective in masking night terror symptoms. Ironically, my sleep clinic records from years earlier contained a written reference to Klonopin. But the doctor who interpreted the report for me never mentioned that the writer had suggested I try this drug.

Years of stagnation finally gave way to rapid progress. At first, taking the recommended dosage of Klonopin left me drained and confused during the day. Why benzodiazepine drugs like Klonopin have this effect will be discussed later. I drastically reduced the dosage myself until I found an acceptable balance between improved sleep and unimpaired daytime performance. The sleep gave me the alertness to begin making sense of the mountain of logs, data, and information that I had collected. And the understandings and adjustments that ensued resulted in the end of my night terror problem and the termination of any further need to take Klonopin.

The Perplexing Night Terror Storms

Although for forty years my bedtime had been anything but peaceful, as I grew older, my Type B Night Terrors became increasingly severe. In the last decade before they ceased, sleeping had become the most intensely tumultuous and physically harmful part of my existence. I am not unique; I was experiencing what many others have experienced. When a night terror victim goes to sleep, the turmoil of his life is just waking up. That turmoil erupts with awesome ferocity very shortly after he or she falls into deep sleep.

The following is typical of most night terror sufferers and is reflective of the symptoms of both Type A and Type B night terrors. Within ten to forty minutes he or she bolts up, sometimes leaping out of bed, eyes wide open, unbelievably frightened, heart pounding, arms flailing, sweating, extremely animated, and usually screaming. The victim is fully asleep yet is exhibiting one of the most intense demonstrations of sheer terror a human being is capable of. After waking, however, he or she usually remembers little or nothing of the episode.

Nothing else known to medical science will cause a person's heart rate to triple in seconds while fast asleep, yet this is what happens. It is an indescribable feeling of terror and panic to such a degree that there have been cases of victims leaping through plate glass windows while having a night terror attack. The victim may have several of these episodes per week and, unless you have experienced one or seen one yourself, the emotional intensity is almost impossible to comprehend. This severity far exceeds what might occur during a nightmare.

Written descriptions of night terror attacks cannot adequately express their intensity. In recent years, several TV shows have broadcast footage of actual attacks that were taped at sleep disorder clinics. Men and women of various ages, who are sleeping soundly one minute, suddenly begin screaming while throwing themselves out of bed and into the air. They kick at the door or the walls, break lamps, and smash furniture in a violent, uncontrolled frenzy that may last up to fifteen minutes. They even sometimes unlock doors and roam around the house. Family members talk to them about going back to bed as if they were awake, but they are not. Usually they return to bed by themselves and remember nothing the next morning.

On the show *20/20*, anchor Hugh Downs showed footage of such an attack as he introduced a television segment about night terrors (March 1996). He then said, "It is a bad dream taken to unbelievable extremes, not a nightmare. In a nightmare the body is in an induced state of paralysis and the person remains in bed until awaking. With night terrors there is no protective paralysis and the victim thrashes, kicks, leaps about, and may leave the house—all without waking up—and will remember nothing of the event the next morning."

The program went on to recount the experiences of several night terror victims. One account was of a young woman, overly tired and sleeping at a friend's house, who had gotten out of bed, crashed through a window and fallen to the street below. She got up, walked back into the house on her own, and was found sleeping on the kitchen floor the next morning. She was bleeding from cuts and was badly bruised—but she remembered nothing!

On a similar program (April 6, 1996), Oprah Winfrey interviewed a middle-aged couple. "I never know when it's going to happen," said the wife. "There seems to be no connection to whether we had a great day or had an argument. But suddenly he grabs or slaps me and threatens me [saying]: 'Why are you here? I hate you. I want you to die!' "

"And what do you have to say about that?" Oprah asked the husband after the camera panned over the stunned audience.

"I don't remember anything," he replied. "I just go to bed and sleep. Then in the morning she tells me I've said those terrible things. I can't understand it. I love my wife and children."

"It's been going on for years," the wife said. "Sometimes several times a week. I'm afraid to go to sleep. I've tried to not take what he says seriously, but after a while it's hard not to. On top of the emotional pain, I'm scared for my physical well-being. I'm never sure what he may do next. He's violent and hateful."

"I love her. I'd never do anything to hurt her," the husband meekly replied. The members of the studio audience, mostly female, shook their heads in disbelief.

"My situation is different," said a young man on the same program. "I'm not violent toward others, but I feel like I'm dying. I scream, 'I can't breathe, I can't breathe!' I leap out of bed, gasping as if for my life. There's no dream. I don't know why I think I'm dying, but I'm terrified that I will. It occurs over and over. I now lock myself in my room. I have videotapes of me jumping on the bed and leaping all over the room. It's like watching a stranger in my body."

Although videos are far more graphic than written accounts of night terror attacks, they still come nowhere near to conveying the unbelievable intensity of what is going on inside the night terror victim's body. The emotional experience is impossible to describe in words or pictures.

The sufferers must be hurting themselves badly, yet they show no signs of pain until the next day. Their fierce, irrational behavior—as if they were fighting off an invisible attacker—appears to be fueled by a huge adrenaline rush brought on by the sheer terror of the moment. But terror of what? Who are the tormenting invisible demons that can cause such wild and bizarre behavior? Why do these incidents have no predictable patterns—sometimes being infrequent for years and then, suddenly, happening several times a week? Doctors do not know, and the victims are no help. Most experts offer vague advice, examples of which can be paraphrased as follows:

- Since they are young, they'll probably grow out of it. It's not uncommon among children.

- It has a lot to do with sleep deprivation. Try not to be over-tired when you go to bed.
- If you are prone to have these, it is better to sleep in your own bed.
- Medication and exercise can generally control the problem.

The symptoms of night terrors have been documented, and the varying severity levels of the condition have been noted. But are these symptoms isolated or widespread? No one really knows, because only recently have a significant number of sufferers been correctly diagnosed. Many cases, perhaps most, remain hidden and undiagnosed. A great number of sufferers probably do not seek medical help and prefer to keep their night terrors a personal or family secret because they are embarrassed to admit that they have the problem. These victims are afraid of being ridiculed for bizarre behavior and/or they fear that what they have to tell will not be believed. On top of this, braving the embarrassment has been pointless for the sufferer. There simply has been little benefit or relief to be found in seeking medical intervention.

As a result, ongoing night terror storms continue to disrupt countless families while the night terror sufferers themselves remain without answers, solutions, or hope. But, thankfully, select writings from other trauma-related scenarios provide valuable insight into some of the mysteries intrinsic to all night terrors.

Chapter 3

Unearthing the Accurate Night Terror Literature

The vast majority of night terror literature is inaccurate in its insistence upon the theory that the condition is genetic in origin. This may be the primary reason professionals have had so little success understanding and treating the malady. Unfortunately, the smattering of articles that deal with extreme psychic trauma preceding the onset of Type B Night Terrors lay buried and ignored within the professional archives. How sad. These articles are filled with information helpful in understanding, diagnosing, and even curing Type B Night Terrors.

Being personally afflicted with Type B Night Terrors for the greater part of my life allowed me to sort through over half a century of conflicting information and then focus on the sparse writings that seemed exceptionally pertinent, conscientious, and insightful. Years later, through assimilating and applying my findings from this valuable research, I was finally able to effectively cure my own night terrors. I then began writing articles on the subject, as well as an earlier draft of this book, in order to begin helping others with what I had learned.

After two years of circulating one of my more lengthy and comprehensive night terror articles among select professional journals, *The California Therapist* accepted and published it in March of 2000. That article was filled with quotations from decades of professional writings that linked the development of Type B Night Terrors to past extreme trauma. There had been nothing tentative or reserved about the writings of these experts. They were sure that Type B Night Terrors were the result of extreme trauma. Unfortunately, most of them went to their graves without successfully impressing their understandings upon their peers. As I discuss elsewhere, it was left for a major recent study to finally validate and prove their findings accurate.

The literature dealing with night terrors among Holocaust survivors was especially fascinating and thorough. Other writings also linked extreme trauma with the onset of Type B Night Terrors. In the studies of those intermittent, rare group-trauma situations, the same connections were made over and over again. While fifty years of literature had documented different times, different people, and entirely different stresses, what remained the same was the conclusion that Type B Night Terrors develop because an individual is exposed to extreme psychic trauma.

The professional community has overlooked this valuable body of work. It has demanded controlled experimentation before it will alter the status quo, and it has been unaware of the fact that in this circumstance, observational research is the only option. The very nature of an accurate laboratory study would be monstrously immoral and highly illegal. A controlled experiment might entail taking 100 infants, 100 toddlers, and 100 school-aged children and mercilessly torturing half of them. Then the tortured children from each group would be compared with the nontortured children for the next decade or so in order that psychological manifestations and sleep disruption could be documented and noted.

Obviously, science cannot set up the conditions needed to conduct such experiments. But, due to the intermittent baseness of the human condition, such studies (after the fact) already do exist. The Nazi death camps, other war-related situations, POW camps, deranged kidnappers, and sadistic caretakers and parents have been providing public and private "laboratories" and multitudes of unfortunate subjects which definitively prove the relationship between extreme trauma and Type B Night Terrors.

Only recently, another group extreme-trauma situation occurred. As we all know, terrorists crashed hijacked commercial airplanes into the World Trade Center Towers and the Pentagon. The towers fell and the Pentagon was damaged. Thousands were killed, badly burned, or otherwise injured in the carnage. Many of the injured witnessed the death of co-workers and friends, or watched people leap to their death from the flaming towers. It's quite possible that in the near future, mental health experts, especially in the New York and Washington areas, might see disrupted sleep, recurring nightmares, or possibly Type B Night Terrors emerge among the survivors. Even family members of those whose loved ones were killed in the disaster may eventually develop sleep and/or anxiety disorders. It is also quite possible that other extreme disasters may still be forthcoming during the troubled times in which we now live.

The nature of the attacks made it very likely that there would soon be reports of sleep disruption among the victims. Less than six months after 9/11, the February 28, 2002, *Orange County* (California) *Register*, along with other national dailies, reported on 350 New York firefighters with stress-related problems. The *Register* wrote that "hundreds of firefighters and emergency medical workers who responded to the World Trade Center attack have reported *nightmares,* sudden anger and other psychological symptoms *so severe that they were taken off active duty.*" (54, p.7)

Simple nightmares would not be severe enough to warrant taking seasoned firefighters off active duty. After all, most parents would not find it necessary to keep their children home from school the day after they've had a simple nightmare. The "nightmares" resulting from 9/11 certainly sound like the extreme-trauma-related and repetitive kind that typify Type B Night Terrors.

Back in 1998, Dr. Ernest Hartmann, one of the most brilliant, thorough, and insightful authorities on sleep and dreaming, had already pointed out the specific and now suddenly pertinent traumatic events that lead to the above types of sleep disorders. He reported: "I have been able to collect long dream series from a number of people who experienced *a trauma such as barely es-*

caping from a fire, or having someone killed next to them. These series clearly show that dreams make connections between the traumatic event and other material." Most disturbingly, Hartmann added, "Clinicians have repeatedly noted that patients with chronic repetitive nightmares resist psychotherapy and seldom benefit from treatment." (27, pp.7, 32)

Conventional treatments for trauma-related repetitive sleep disorders have been totally ineffective for far too long. However, interest in finding solutions is growing and will continue to grow as the media reports on the symptoms of more and more 9/11 victims. In contrast to the Holocaust scenario, the World Trade Center bombing is so well documented and the time differential between the event and the emergence of symptoms is so short that the cause and effect relationship between the trauma and the resultant psychological aberrations is direct and undeniable. This particular group-trauma situation clearly demonstrates the link between the traumatic event and the development of Type B Night Terrors, repetitive nightmares, and other psychological manifestations.

The profusion of victims evidencing trauma-related disorders as a result of the terrorist attacks is growing daily. For example, an astounding unforeseen repercussion surprised medical professionals on May 2, 2002, when it was reported that "nearly 90 percent of New York City schoolchildren were suffering from post traumatic stress six months after Sept. 11. In the 1.1 million pupil public school system, an estimated 75,000 children likely showed six or more symptoms of post-traumatic stress. 24 percent had problems sleeping and 17 percent had nightmares."

The tragic events of 9/11 and their consequences, both immediate and long lasting, serve to further substantiate decades of work by a small body of brilliant researchers. These exceptional, intuitive, and conscientious professionals have carefully examined the victims of past atrocities after the fact, documenting and exposing some of the causal factors that are essential to the development of Type B Night Terrors. Although the significance of their work has been largely ignored, their findings should soon begin to receive more attention. This is due to the fact that the writings of those who have supported the theory that Type B Night Terrors are trauma-related have finally been proved accurate in the groundbreaking *Journal of the American Medical Association* article mentioned earlier. Charles B. Nemeroff's *JAMA* article is significant because it documents what is probably the most important laboratory study ever done on the subject of child abuse, and because it gives compelling physical evidence that anxiety disorders in adults, such as Type B Night Terrors, can definitely be traced to chemical changes in the brain resulting from extreme abuse.

It appears that professionals have been polarized as a result of the old debate over genetic versus environmental factors in the etiology of psychiatric disorders. But the *JAMA* article, at the very least, should result in some kind of consensus and direction to the benefit of all victims of child abuse, including those who suffer from Type B Night Terrors, by means of findings such as the following regarding nongenetic but psychological and physiological factors:

"Considerable evidence from a variety of studies suggest a preeminent roll of early adverse experiences in the development of mood and anxiety disorders . . . Our findings suggest that hypothalamic-pituitary-adrenal axis and autonomic nervous system hyperactivity, presumably due to CRF (corticotropin-releasing factor) hypersecretion, is a persistent consequence of childhood abuse that may contribute to the diathesis for adulthood psychopathological conditions." (4, p.592, 593) The article also states that CRF produces psychological and behavioral changes, disruption of sleep being one of them.

"Childhood abuse also predisposes to the development of anxiety disorders in adulthood, including panic disorder and generalized anxiety disorder. In addition, post traumatic stress disorder (PTSD) may be a direct consequence of childhood abuse, and moreover, such trauma early in life also appears to increase an individual's risk of developing PTSD in response to other traumas in adulthood." (4, p. 593)

"Severe stress early in life is associated with persistent sensitization of the pituitary-adrenal and autonomic stress response, which, in turn, is likely related to an increased risk for adult psychopathological conditions. This is the first human study to report persistent changes in stress reactivity in adult survivors of early trauma." (4, p. 596)

To clarify these findings in layman's terms, the study examined adult women who had experienced documented childhood trauma. Advances in science allowed for detailed brain chemistry analysis of these women, and it was found that nervous system damage had occurred. Their bodies were producing an overabundance of chemicals that we now know play a role in many mood and anxiety disorders. Prior to this study most of these disorders and conditions were attributed to genetics. This first-of-its-kind study definitively proves that many of these maladies are the latent biological result of extreme childhood trauma.

The *JAMA* study has finally confirmed what the late Dr. Leo Eitinger had already figured out decades ago. He himself had been interned in Auschwitz. After the war he had devoted the rest of his life to studying and documenting the post-captivity physiological and psychological problems of his fellow survivors. While Eitinger is the most highly qualified voice ever to speak on this subject, you would have to be a night terror sufferer yourself to perceive the absolute brilliance and flawless precision of his writings. He was able to come to understand and express the intricacies of this subject on a level that few have approached. He paid particular attention to those who were imprisoned in the Nazi death camps as children. He forcefully and repeatedly pointed out that the stress of the camps, not genetic factors, had caused changes at the biological level. Dr. Eitinger wrote, "It is obvious that experiences of the traumatic magnitude we are dealing with here, must act almost independently of the premorbid personality." (11, p. 169)

Eitinger and Schwarz stated: "However, some psychiatrists still hold the view that psychological symptoms following exposure to stressful situations occur only in predisposed individuals. . . . This form of reasoning stems from the ignorance induced by an almost total absence of knowledge of the late social, occupational and psychological effects in individuals who have survived situations involving great physical danger and psychological stress . . . When individuals are subjected to a prolonged threat to their survival, the evidence suggests that pre-existing personality characteristics resulting from inherited and earlier environmental experiences are replaced by *a universal and basic biological reaction.*" (9, pp.215-217)

Dr. Eitinger observed that all the Auschwitz survivors developed Type B Night Terrors. The condition was especially severe among the children. Long before the *JAMA* study, he knew that something was happening at the biological level. In determining the guidelines for what was later termed "concentration camp syndrome," Eitinger stated that he and other psychiatrists "excluded nightmares and anxiety because [these] were present in *all* the interviewed survivors." (12, p.479) As mentioned earlier, although he used the term "nightmare," in reading the brunt of Dr. Eitinger's writings, it is indisputable that he was discussing Type B Night Terror symptoms being experienced by concentration camp survivors. There is a distinction in his writings between concentration camp survivors and other Jews who survived the Holocaust but were not interned in camps. The incidence of Type B Night Terrors among the latter group was substantially reduced.

In trying to determine which manifestations and symptoms resulted from the more lengthy, severe, and brutal treatment of prisoners, Eitinger could not use Type B Night Terrors and anxiety as criteria. This was because even those prisoners who had a relatively less traumatic incarceration and were liberated after a very short internment in the camps suffered from Type B Night Terrors and anxiety with varying degrees of severity and frequency. The trauma was so extreme at Auschwitz, even for those who had relatively less exposure to it, that Type B Night Terrors and anxiety became universal among the survivors.

On the other hand, symptoms such as diminished mental capacity, a limited ability to concentrate, and badly deteriorated memorization skills were found only in those prisoners whose internment was lengthy and extremely brutal. Before the war, many of these mentally damaged people had been intelligent, competent, highly educated individuals. Eitinger knew that extreme stress had caused some kind of breakdown at the biological level and that the severity of this breakdown was in proportion to the intensity of the stress and the length of time the individual was exposed to it. Furthermore, he concluded that even a short period of extreme stress (such as at Auschwitz) was sufficient to cause all the survivors to develop Type B Night Terrors and anxiety.

Another Holocaust researcher, Dr. Chodoff, arrived at the same conclusion and wrote: "When one considers the intensity of the stress undergone by these patients, there seems little necessity to postulate any pre-existing personality weakness or predisposition. Any man can break if the stress is severe enough. . . . Possibly, psychodynamic psychiatry has gone too far in its at least implied insistence that every state of emotional illness must result from the impact of a trauma on a personality somehow predisposed to react adversely to the trauma; cases of the kind described here must be taken into account before such explanations can be regarded as universal." (15, p.327)

Other researchers looked at different life-threatening situations and noted the same kinds of Type B Night Terrors that emerged among Holocaust survivors. Leopold and Dillon wrote: "The same failure of repression has been noted by the authors among survivors of Nazi concentration camps. . . . The authors feel that the psychiatric community as a whole has failed to recognize the significance of the nature of accident itself, and particularly its suddenness, in the development of the post-traumatic states. For reasons not entirely clear, it appears more usual to regard the pre-accident personality as a major factor, and to relegate the accident itself to the role of a mere triggering circumstance which sets off an illness considered almost certain to have occurred in any case." (16, pp.919, 920) Here the authors clearly indicate that the event, the accident (trauma) itself, produces the effects if the stress is severe enough and prolonged enough. This shows that predisposition is not a necessary factor.

In 1973, Fisher, Kahn, Edwards and Davis also attributed Type B Night Terrors to trauma. "We have seen a 40-year-old survivor of the concentration camp, Auschwitz, who, from the ages of 11 to 14, sustained overwhelming trauma and developed severe night terrors during which he somnambulistically acted out scenes of persecution." (14, p. 96)

Dr. Marshall stated: "In my experience, the post traumatic syndrome is the most common clinical situation with which night terrors in adults are associated." (8, p. 295) And Dr. Neylan and associates wrote: "The nightmare appears to be the primary domain of sleep disturbance related to exposure to war zone traumatic stress." (17, p. 929)

Type B Night Terror manifestations developing from diverse scenarios are even more pronounced in the cases which Susan Knapp recounted about the children of the 1976 Chowchilla, California, kidnapping. In a small town about 150 miles southeast of San Francisco, three masked men boarded a school bus, abducted the driver plus twenty-six children at gunpoint, and then herded the terrified captives into two vans. Eleven hours later, the driver and children—ages five to fourteen—were removed from the vans and buried six feet underground in a small, poorly ventilated moving van. They were entombed for the next sixteen hours, slowly overheating and nearly suffocating to death. Even though the bus driver ultimately found a way for them to escape, the children had endured extreme psychic trauma during the entire twenty-seven-hour ordeal.

As mentioned earlier, Knapp reported that night terrors could develop in a child of any age and that the children's "dreams" contained similar content to the night terror "dreams" of adults suffering from traumatic war neurosis. She also wrote: "The fact that so many of the children of Chowchilla suffered from night terrors *definitely* points to the emergence of this disorder in response to psychic trauma." (5, pp.185,192) She concurred with the previously mentioned writers when stating, "Even in normal individuals, when there is significant trauma there will be a break-down of defenses, and night terrors might emerge." (5, p.192) Knapp's observations about Chowchilla are the bedrock of her bold assertions. She was able to dismiss prevailing theory and concentrate on and draw conclusions based on what she saw.

In another article about Chowchilla, Dr. Lenore Terr stated that: "In studies of adults from concentration camps, the battle-field, or peacetime stress, all types of dreams found in the Chow-chilla children have been described." (18, p.594) She implored her fellow professionals to take a good hard look at this particular scenario: "Few, if any opportunities like the Chowchilla kidnap-ping have presented themselves for study of the effect of a psychic trauma upon an entire group." (18, p. 549)

While the astute writings of the people listed above were ig-nored, genetic theories were not. Dr. Kales wrote: "Night terrors also may occur in multiple family members. Hallstrom (1972) re-ported three affected individuals and three consecutive generations, and suggested an autosomal dominant pattern of heritability." (19, p.111)

Because we now know that children who are severely abused oftentimes become abusive parents themselves, we clearly under-stand that the generational patterns of abuse-related anxiety dis-orders are environmental and not hereditary. Dr. Charles Carlson and Dr. David White were thinking along these lines when they wrote: "Presently, it is not clear that night terrors have a genetic component to their etiology, because it is just as likely that the families in which night terrors occur are those families who do not cope effectively with stress or anxiety." (20, p.461)

But many went along with the heredity theories about Type B Night Terrors despite very strong evidence that the condition was unrelated to genetics. Robinson and associates stated that 94 per-cent of Holocaust survivors went on to have children and that on top of this, 69 percent married other Holocaust survivors (21, p.313) This meant that if night terrors were tied to genetics, there would be a substantial number of offspring who had both parents contributing to the genetic likelihood of developing them. If 94 percent of a group suffering from a genetic condition that is passed on through heredity went on to have offspring, there would be a virtual explosion of night terror cases among this next generation, especially in Israel. Although evidence of such an explosion of second-generation night terror cases would be apparent and easily documented, there was no such phenomenon. In fact, studies have shown just the opposite. Dr. Paul Schmolling stated, "There was no evidence that the traumatic experience of survivors generated psychopathology in the offspring." (22, p.118) Robinson and associates came to a similar conclusion: "Despite the apparent mental suffering after the war and today, Holocaust survivors have managed to cope and to adjust. Most of them were absorbed and settled well in Israel. They succeeded in raising stable families with a warm atmosphere." (21, p. 314) Thousands of offspring were produced by a group composed almost exclusively of people who were suffering from a supposed genetically transferred condition, yet these thousands of offspring show no more incidence of the condition than the general population at large.

Almost all of the *JAMA* findings were already in the professional literature. But more important, the latest science explains the reasons behind the documented observations of the past. For example, in 1990 Dr. Jules Rosen and associates wrote: "The group of survivors who had frequent [Type B Night Terrors] had spent more time in camps." (23, p.65) *JAMA* reported that, "The magnitude of abuse is correlated with the severity [of the disorders developed in adulthood]." (4, p.592) These studies emphasize the importance of duration and severity as factors.

Dr. Jules Rosen and associates also noted that "impaired sleep and frequent [Type B Night Terrors] are considerable problems even forty-five years after liberation." (23, p. 65) An article from *Newsweek* magazine pertaining to the high school shootings in Littleton, Colorado, stated: "The dark side of the zero-to-3 movement, which emphasizes the huge potential for learning during this period, is that the young brain also is extra vulnerable to hurt in the first years of life. A child who suffers repeated 'hits' of stress—abuse, neglect, terror—experiences physical changes to the brain." (24, p.32)

After giving a list of symptoms, Eitinger wrote: "This summary of the symptoms does not recount much about the patients' sufferings and hopelessness, but does show how little has been achieved for these people by treatment. All these patients have been under psychotherapy for several years." (11, p.170) Serious, trauma-related brain damage, as documented by *JAMA,* supports the *Newsweek* conclusions and also explains why professional intervention has proven unsuccessful for so long.

In a 1973 experiment, Dr. Fisher and his associates were able to induce artificial night terror attacks that were as severe as spontaneous episodes by simply sounding a loud buzzer while the sufferer was in stage four sleep. (14, p.78) What did a buzzer have to do with the triggering of night terror attacks? The *JAMA* report explained that one of the negative consequences of excessive CRF hypersecretion is a "potentiation of acoustic startle responses." (4, p.593) In other words, an overabundance of CRF—corticotropin-releasing factor—amplifies human reaction to unexpected noise. That is why Dr. Fisher was able to induce artificial night terror attacks with a buzzer.

And finally, *JAMA* found that the brain changes caused by early extreme trauma could be reversed by administering the antidepressants paroxetine (Paxil) and reboxetine. (4, p.596) By random experimentation, drugs similar to these were found to mask night terror symptoms years ago. Thanks to this study, we now understand how and why these drugs had some positive effect on Type B Night Terror sufferers. In the past, few people suspected that these drugs were actually working to counter trauma-related brain damage.

The quotations above are only a very small sampling of the thousands of pages of professional writings stating that Type B Night Terrors are definitely a product of exposure to extreme trauma. Overlooking this valuable literature has resulted in a huge potential for healing going unrealized for decades. The beginning of effective treatment was and is dependent upon an understanding of the link between extreme trauma and Type B Night Terrors. Collectively, astute writers had exhaustively explored, thoroughly explained and definitively documented this link decades ago, long before the *JAMA* study proved it.

Chapter 4

Type A Night Terrors

Since true childhood Type A Night Terrors are far more common than trauma-related Type B Night Terrors, I would guess that most people are reading this book in order to find out more about the childhood Type A variety. While it is important to clearly comprehend the difference between the two conditions, it behooves all those interested in Type A to become knowledgeable about Type B, and vice versa.

Type A Night Terrors involve no child abuse or extreme trauma, no serious psychopathology, no brain damage, no troubled mind, and no long-lasting effects. What else do we know about these terrors? Although there are disagreements about actual percentages, the following 1991 statement by Dr. Garland and Dr. Smith is universally supported and accepted. They said, "Night terrors and somnambulism, considered to be disorders of arousal, are estimated to occur in about 3 percent of children. Although research on the occurrence and natural history is limited, in one study, 36 percent of childhood night terror cases persisted into adolescence." (25, p.553)

Although most researchers list the estimated occurrence of night terrors in children at around 3 percent, they list the number of these cases that persist into adolescence at less than 36 percent. Additionally, the percentage of cases that continue into adulthood is reported to be small. Dr. Joyce Kales and associates stated that, "Night terrors typically begin in childhood or early adolescence and are usually 'outgrown' by the end of adolescence." (26, p.1214) As we have already seen, this basic truth is repeated throughout almost all of the reliable night terror literature.

However, the statistics are highly misleading. All estimated percentages are inherently unreliable because the numbers reflect only the reported cases. Night terrors in general are an underreported, "closet" condition. One only has to bring the subject up at a PTA meeting or other large gathering to see that there are many people who personally know of someone who has experienced this kind of sleep disorder.

The numbers in almost all studies reflect the fact that Type A Night Terrors are relatively common in children and that the majority of young people will ultimately outgrow the condition. Therefore, for the purposes of this chapter, the actual percentages are far less important than the fact stated above. More important, the percentages make little difference to the sufferer or to the one who must watch helplessly as he or she thrashes about in the grip of a night terror episode. Therefore, the following chapters will be useful not only to night terror sufferers and professionals in the field; they will also expose caregivers to increased understandings, workable strategies, and viable suggestions as to the most effective steps to take in dealing with night terrors.

Parents are often quite upset by the child's apparent distress, as Susan Knapp states. It is common for parents to have experienced unbelievable agony in the process of simply trying to find out what is wrong with their child. Many general practitioners are uninformed about the condition. The veracity of what the parent is telling the doctor is often questioned, dismissed, or completely ignored. In pursuing this with other professionals, parents have run into either more of the same or, sometimes, questions directed at the parents which constitute veiled accusations of abuse. Those parents who are coming forward looking for help usually are not the ones who are abusing their children. They are most likely investigating the simple, innocent Type A Night Terror condition. It is the parents who are not coming forward who should cause us to question their lack of concern for their children, as well as their possible complicity in causing the ailment.

After what usually amounts to an exhaustive, lengthy, and frustrating process, some parents may finally find a professional who has at least heard of the condition. They are then told that the medical community does not understand much about night terrors, but that the condition probably has something to do with genetics and that the child will most likely outgrow it. At this point, despair and hopelessness are added to the caregiver's frustration. He or she is forced to conclude that there is no help and there are no answers.

Those professionals whose own children have experienced Type A Night Terrors are not nearly so nonchalant. Dr. Dement wrote: "I can remember my own daughter terrified and whimpering in the night. Even though I was somewhat of an expert on night terrors, it was very difficult not to panic myself." (1, p.212) What sort of panic do parents experience who are not experts on night terrors? Even for an observer who is not related to the child, a night terror attack is a very difficult thing to watch.

While recent discoveries clarify much of the mystery surrounding Type B Night Terrors, they shed very little light on the Type A variety. Even though no one is absolutely certain what causes Type A Night Terrors to begin and then just as suddenly to end, the literature hints that the condition results from an overreaction by a child's fledgling emotional system misinterpreting rather mundane environmental stresses. If this is true, then it would make sense that an unexplained resolution would occur when the child reached an age of more advanced cerebral comprehension with correspondingly elevated association skills. Some of the more insightful Type B Night Terror literature dealing with the Chowchilla, California, kidnapping points to the above as a possible explanation for Type A Night Terrors. A simple exaggerated fear of the mundane that gets resolved as the child matures emotionally and cerebrally certainly justifies the medical community's casual regard for this condition and might also explain why Type A Night Terrors "typically disappear without treatment." (7, p.99)

Dr. Lenore Terr noted that not all of the children involved in the Chowchilla kidnapping developed Type B Night Terrors. She wrote: "While evaluating the Chowchilla children, I rated their ability to verbalize their feelings. Seven children were particularly nonverbal about emotion. Six children experienced only unremembered terror dreams. Six of the seven Chowchilla youngsters who never fully acquired the ability to verbalize emotions, *like toddlers,* dreamed dreams for which no words could later be found. Without words, there was only nameless terror." (18, p.597) Dr. Terr observed that the same level of stress did not exceed the breaking point of the emotionally verbal children but did exceed the breaking point of the emotionally nonverbal children. Her study confirmed that the age of the individual is important in determining how intense the stress must be in order to produce Type B Night Terrors.

Susan Knapp insightfully explained the mechanics of Type B Night Terrors. She wrote: "In the night terror the child recreates the original trauma, but then, by awakening, is able to gain a measure of mastery, in that escape is now possible." (5, p.185) This is both fascinating and accurate. Videotape of Type B Night Terror victims shows them apparently fighting back against some invisible attacker. In the case of the Holocaust survivors, POWs, and tortured infants, fighting back at the time of the actual trauma was impossible. With infants it was not physically possible to fight back, and with Holocaust survivors and POWs, fighting back meant death. In my own Type B Night Terror attacks I would always leap up screaming and "escape" just prior to the onset of the most painful torture. The Type B Night Terror recreation substitutes a fictitious ending for the most traumatic event of the individual's life. The actions during such a night terror attack are a futile attempt to rewrite an ending that has already taken place, alter personal history, change an outcome, finally "escape" or master a situation that was out of one's control at the time. The content of my own night terrors left me with no doubt that Susan Knapp was correct. Others have arrived at similar conclusions.

Dr. Ernest Hartmann concurred with Susan Knapp and even used similar wording when talking about a group of researchers who, after extensive study, concluded that "dreams play a role in mastering stress." (27, p.125) Stresses that we are not aware of when awake or that are too painful to deal with can safely be dealt with and possibly mastered while dreaming. Hartmann wrote that: "The connections [made during dreams] appear to be guided principally by the emotions or emotional concerns of the dreamer." (27, p.7) He also stated that dreams help us to address "an emotional concern of which we may not have been entirely aware," (27, p.10) or an emotional issue that may be "blocked off and cannot be assessed by waking thought." (27 p.181) Bear in mind that when talking about Type A Night Terrors, stress and trauma are relative terms. There has been no genuine extreme trauma in these cases. Only the child perceives it as such. Hartmann himself explains that "trauma is not necessarily the same thing for different people." (27, p.34)

Of course, cases grounded in genuine extreme trauma can be tremendously helpful in understanding the mechanics of mastering stress through dreams and nightmares. Conscious as well as unconscious behaviors make perfect sense to us because we are aware of the entire trauma scenario and history. For example, in another article about the Chowchilla kidnapping, Dr. Terr wrote: "When the kidnappers filled gas tanks of the vans with gasoline, Allison, 10, who is asthmatic, believed that she was being asphyxiated. . . . One year after the kidnapping Allison's mother related, 'the new car makes her go crazy. She says, in the back of the car it doesn't get cool enough. She huffs and puffs and says she can't breathe.' Long after the kidnapping, fear of further trauma continued to operate as a force behind the fears of the mundane from which 21 of the 23 children suffered." (28, p.16) Even the older children displayed "fears of the mundane."

I believe the above observations play a role in the onset, manifestations, and resolution of Type A Night Terrors. With very few emotional defenses in place, it would only take minimal stress to cause extreme emotional fear in infants or toddlers. An infant or toddler who was entwined in the crib blankets and suffocating might from that point on begin to experience nocturnal panic attacks in which the original trauma is re-created. Then, the acting out of an escape might appear to evidence all the intensity, adrenaline, and emotional power of a Type B Night Terror attack because the urgency and seriousness of the stress would seem as real to the child's psyche as an actual extreme trauma would be to an adult. This might explain why the less serious Type A Night Terror symptoms and trauma-related Type B Night Terror symptoms appear the same when experienced by children. But there has been no real extreme trauma in Type A cases. This type of night terror—nonserious, shallow rooted, non-psychologically aberrant, and self-resolving—could simply be a product of an exaggerated "fear of the mundane" being played out in a seemingly real way in the child's sleeping subconscious. All this really means is that the child may be fearfully reacting to something that an adult would probably find fairly unthreatening or commonplace.

For those parents who have observed their own children in the throes of a night terror episode, I'm sure that this scenario does not sound far-fetched. If the child is recreating the unbelievable fright experienced as an infant when entwined in a blanket (or something else), unable to free himself and in sheer panic, it would explain what the parents or other caregivers are observing. The bulging eyes, profuse sweating, screaming, flailing arms, and a heart thumping hard enough almost to burst right out of the chest are symptoms consistent with the ones an adult displays when his sleeping subconscious is reliving or re-creating a genuine traumatic experience.

The big difference of course is in the origins of this unbelievably intense panic. In the case of a Type A Night Terror sufferer, it was caused by something completely benign and innocent. In the case of a Type B Night Terror victim, it was caused by something heinous and/or malicious. However, the panic experienced by the sufferer is just as real to him/her in both cases. The infant's lack of life experience and fledgling emotional defense system turn this relatively minor stress into the most fearful and devastating event of his or her young life. This indicates that it is possible to trace even Type A Night Terrors to nongenetic causes.

Therefore, I believe there is a plausible nongenetic explanation for why Type A Night Terrors begin, and also for why the panic expressed by the child is so intense and animated. But, the thing I find most interesting is how well the resolution of Type A Night Terrors seems to fit. Why do these cases resolve themselves in late childhood or early adolescence? No one really knows. But, if it were true that Type A Night Terrors disappear according to a set timetable, there would be little you could do to speed the process along. I simply do not believe that the condition just disappears by itself or that the resolution process is arbitrary or haphazard. Late childhood and early adolescence are when children have already passed through various mental and emotional developmental stages. Additionally, some are given responsibility for younger siblings, exposed to infants at the houses of relatives or friends, or begin babysitting the infant children of family or neighbors. I strongly suspect that in such cases the Type A Night Terror victim's contact with the infant can lead to observations and mental associations that affirm the mundane nature of the trauma that has been haunting the subconscious.

For instance, suppose a near-suffocation from being trapped in a blanket is the root trauma that has been replayed in the sufferer's subconscious for all these years. He or she may observe an infant sibling momentarily trapped in a blanket, dash to help, and without even realizing it, make a subconscious connection that affirms how truly benign the events of his or her own night terror really were. After the subconscious makes this connection there is no further reason for it to "recreate the original trauma" and thereby try to "gain a measure of mastery." (5 p.185) Mastery has just been gained, but not even the sufferer is aware of what has happened. Therefore, the child who has been plagued by Type A Night Terrors for many years may all of a sudden, without explanation, be completely free of the condition. The symptoms may

never return. This is but one example of the many types of reve-
latory experiences children can have as they mature that can help
to resolve their Type A Night Terror problems.

Children have no awareness of what is true or real as perceived by an adult. At three, a child screams in fright when an
older sibling jumps out from behind the door, when at six, the
same child may laugh. Shadows, cries in the night, strangers in
the park, stories in children's books or movies can trigger fear
and nightmares. To children there may be no explanation for
their night apparitions. Accepting that the visions are real to
them, giving them validation, and assisting them to acquire
power over their own thoughts are all helpful to a healthy recovery. Therapeutic techniques such as drawing the night images, or
hearing stories of overcoming the "meanies," or "talking it out"
can be very helpful and may even overcome the bad moments
(therapeutic metaphors). Debriefing a child's real or fantasy experiences (explained in detail later), particularly if the child perceives
them as negative, remains critical to linguistic development, emotional security, thought processing, problem solving, and behavioral modeling. (35, p.158) Such interactions between caretakers
and children may be beneficial in the process of resolving childhood sleep disturbances.

Developmentally, a child at four still has difficulty separating
fantasy from reality. He or she cannot answer the question
"What if . . ." Indeed, primitive reasoning is only beginning between the ages of four and seven and is characterized by children
acting as if they are certain that what they "know" is true.
Children lack the ability to give a logical explanation regarding
night terrors. This is what Piaget called the intuitive versus the
logical stage. The child may suffer from night terrors, nightmares, or bad dreams simply from upset feelings over nontrau-
matic mundane events that often go undetected by loved ones.
However, the highly upsetting experiences during these sleep disturbances can be separated from similar real-life occurrences because no actual severe trauma or abuse has taken place. Yet,

caretakers may be worried or not aware of ways to debrief their child's terror.

Piaget pointed out that for many children the age of abstraction, or critical reason, required for sophisticated awareness doesn't arrive until around thirteen years. Often, even adults cannot explain their own nightmares, and show fascination when dreams are discussed. Indeed, many developmental professionals believe there are numerous adults who do not ever gain such skills. (35, p.38) Between seven and thirteen, experiences begin to ground the child in reality. This explains why Type A Night Terrors in children usually cease around this time. All of this points to the necessity of determining the degree of emotional, mental, and behavioral safety in a child's environment in order to detect Type A versus Type B Night Terrors.

Dr. Hartmann, while concurring with Piaget, explained even deeper aspects of children's dreams and nightmares. He wrote: "Almost all children have occasional nightmares, usually involving a theme such as being chased, at some point in their lives (most frequently at age 4 to 6). I believe we can understand these dreams as picturing or contextualizing the inevitable vulnerability of a small child in a world run by larger, much more powerful creatures—adults. (27, p.50) [Dreams] recreate the perceptual world of the dreamer. (p.212) Nightmares are frequently reported though it may not be clear in detail exactly what was experienced by the child. (p.214) In general these dreams usually deal in some way with anxieties and conflicts present in the child's life, sometimes relating to external traumatic events but frequently combining these with the inevitable conflicts or characteristics of a child's developmental phase. In other words, when there is no specific external trauma, dreams and nightmares usually deal with such things as the child's vulnerability." (p. 216) These nightmares, as well as Type A Night Terrors, will usually disappear as the child matures and moves out of particular developmental phases. They self-resolve as the child passes through various stages of vulnerability, conflict, and anxiety. As the waking perceptual world of the child expands, the subconscious fears and nightmares diminish.

This is in sharp contrast to the child who is experiencing Type B Night Terrors. The past events that cause trauma-related night terrors are too extreme ever to be explained away by common daily observations or to be simply outgrown. These events are so traumatic that even the sufferers who know exactly what the trauma entailed cannot come to terms with this horror in spite of years of psychotherapy. The childhood survivors of Auschwitz, who knew precisely which real-life events led to the development of their Type B Night Terrors, are clear examples.

As we now know, severe chemical brain changes have taken place in these individuals. It will necessitate far more than making simple maturational, cerebral, and emotional connections for Type B Night Terrors to go away. These complicated solutions will be explored in a later chapter.

Dr. Hartmann attempted to give a picture of trauma-related mental damage when writing: "If we think of the mind as a net in the concrete sense of a fishnet or a piece of woven cloth, we can think of trauma as a kind of tear in the net." (27, p.122) Hartmann, like Eitinger, discovered that these trauma-related "tears" are highly resistant to mending. Hartmann wrote: "In children, play also becomes repetitive and stuck at such times. And, in fact, psychotherapy frequently does not help greatly either. Clinicians have repeatedly noted that patients with established PTSD and chronic repetitive nightmares resist psychotherapy and seldom benefit from treatment." (27, p.32)

But at least we can understand the patterns and logical manifestations that are side effects associated with a documented trauma. For example, in Dr. Terr's study, it was relatively easy to figure out why Allison experienced such an exaggerated "fear of the mundane." Smelling even the faintest exhaust fumes while sitting in the backseat of a car made this little girl "go crazy" with panic while awake. The smell reminded her of the kidnapping. But bear in mind, this ten-year-old girl was verbal, and the situation that caused her panic was well documented. Both the parents and the therapist understood the obvious connections to the kidnapping.

Suppose instead that the child was nonverbal, and suppose also that no one was aware of the situation that had caused her panic. Both the caregivers and the therapist would be baffled as to why this child went "crazy" with panic when simply seated in the back of the car. No one would have been able to make any logical connection between the smell of gas and Allison's panic attack. We understand this panic in Allison's case because all the information we have puts everyone comfortably inside the child's mind.

I suggest that the parents/caregivers of children suffering from night terrors keep an understanding of the above in the back of their minds. If they understand that in the throes of the night terror attack the child might actually be reacting to "fears of the mundane," then they themselves will have an easier time maintaining their own composure. Rather than watch a child panic, and then panic themselves, they need to consider some of the information above. This is difficult for any parent faced with the actual situation. *But, understanding beforehand that this could simply be an overreaction to something quite benign could prove helpful and calming to caregivers. They could merely be reacting to the fact that they cannot get comfortably inside their child's mind.*

If you could crawl inside your child's mind, you would probably find the same comfort and understanding that Allison's parents got from knowing her situation. Unfortunately, it is not always possible to do that. But if we assume that the child might be acting out of a fear of the mundane, the situation becomes much easier to deal with. Since the great majority of children with night terrors outgrow the condition, the odds are that a highly animated overreaction to some mundane event is exactly what you are witnessing.

You would be far more relaxed if you knew for a fact that the child had been entwined in a blanket early in life, and was merely reenacting the panic from that episode when entering deep sleep.

How much calmer would you be if you were sure that he or she would eventually resolve this satisfactorily and never experience night terrors again?

Parents/caregivers of children suffering from Type A Night Terrors need to understand as much as they can about fears of the mundane. Because of children's limited life experience and fledgling emotional development, the fear they are experiencing and expressing is 100 percent real even though the reason for this fear is not. That is, as judged by an adult, there would seem insufficient reason for children to be so frightened by such an unintimidating stimulus. But they do not see it this way. They are as frightened of this mundane stimulus as an adult would be if faced with a life-and-death situation.

Chapter 5

Diagnosing and Alleviating Type A Night Terrors

This chapter speaks primarily to parents/caregivers who have provided or are concerned about providing a safe, loving environment for children. All people make mistakes, but there is a difference between very abusive and relatively healthy caregivers. Indeed, we must distinguish between those caregivers who cherish children and those who, because of their own mental or emotional illnesses, create a "war zone" in their own homes.

A mistake is accidental and can be corrected without serious damage. An example would be punishing a child and then discovering that another child caused the problem. A healthy parent would apologize to the punished child, sit down with both children, talk over the problem, and indicate what steps will be taken the next time. The unhealthy parent might continue to punish the first child because of feeling foolish for being wrong, or might pass it off as his/her right to do anything to the child because the child belongs to the parent, or hit both children for getting in the way, or say nothing, hoping that the first child won't notice.

This chapter assumes you are one of the healthy parents/caregivers and care deeply about your child. Just as was true with my own case, you'll find that a consummately interested, open-minded novice who is passionately committed to gaining understanding will often be more effective than a busy practitioner who must divide his or her time and attention among numerous patients. As you gather information on night terrors, part of your job is to insist that any professional you work with will listen to your views and partner with you in helping your child through his/her early life.

Parents have to become the experts on their children's night terror problems. Otherwise, there's a 99 percent chance that the condition will be misdiagnosed and mistreated. I'll walk you through the relatively simple steps you need to take in order to become the most qualified expert on the subject of your child's condition.

How does a parent tell if a child is experiencing Type A rather than Type B Night Terrors? As repeatedly stated, the odds are in the parent's favor. The overwhelming majority of childhood night terror cases are Type A; these will resolve themselves in or before adolescence. Only a small minority of the night terror cases experienced by children are rooted in extreme psychic trauma. Initially, the child's history will be the greatest help in making this assessment.

As mentioned earlier, in her 1997 study dealing with impaired sleep among abused children, Dr. Carol Glod found that re-experiencing their abuse while asleep caused recurring distressing dreams. (10, p. 1236) But she also found that "physical abuse appears to exert a more deleterious effect on sleep than did sexual abuse." (10, p.1236)

Looking only for prior physical abuse as a cause for sleep disorders, rather than both physical and sexual abuse, dramatically narrows down the possibilities. Although sexual abuse will lead to other psychological problems, sleep disturbances are not the most common among them. Dr. Glod's surprise discovery that sleep disturbances were more prevalent in children who had been physically abused than in those who had been sexually abused is very helpful in determining if a child is suffering from Type A Night Terrors or not.

If a child was born directly to a set of emotionally stable parents who *wanted the child,* and who *cared* for the child almost *exclusively,* then the chances of the child suffering from trauma-related Type B Night Terrors are *small. There is also no need to start thinking about the relatives or babysitters the child was left with during infancy.* Normally well-adjusted people with average backgrounds, who deal relatively well with stress and anger, simply do not beat and torture infants. That kind of brutality is rare. Such extreme abuse would almost have to be premeditated and deliberate, and usually would be indicative of some kind of sick, lifelong hostility an individual is projecting onto the infant. It's beyond what we normally think of as child abuse. And fortunately natural parents, except in Munchausen by proxy syndrome cases, rarely perpetrate this kind of intense malice on their own children. (People with Munchausen pretend to care about their children while they abuse or harm them or make them sick in order to satisfy a distorted need for self-importance.)

In summary, check for:

• Physical or emotional abuse
• Unknown history
• History of mental or emotional abuse in a major caretaker

If your background assessment falls positively within the guidelines above, then the next step is to begin carefully monitoring and documenting everything related to the child's sleep disruption. If, however, the child was adopted, in a foster home, or not with the natural parents during infancy, a more complicated evaluation is called for. (Those issues will be dealt with in chapter 7, "Clarifying The Diagnosis.") In those cases, the chance that such a child is suffering from the serious, trauma-related Type B Night Terrors increases over those in the natural parent group. Those who are relatively sure that they are dealing with Type A Night Terrors should buy a large spiralbound notebook and begin keeping notes and a log.

The Notes and Log

The first section should be a quick overview of the child's background from the hospital of birth to the present. Next, you should write down everything you remember about the night terrors themselves. At what age did they begin? How frequent or severe have they been? How long has it been going on? Have the symptoms gotten worse? Approximately how many episodes are there per month? Is there screaming? If the child has speech, do the same words consistently accompany the night terror attacks? If he/she is not yet verbal, do the same actions consistently accompany the attacks? How long do they last?

Describe the attack. Is the child sweating, very animated or crying? Are eyes wide open? Is the heart pounding? Does the child wake up during the attack or remember anything about it the next morning? Are there multiple episodes or just one? Do they always occur within the first hour after falling asleep? Did the child nap during the day? How physical or stressful a day was it for him/her? Did the child run around wildly with siblings or friends just prior to bedtime, or did he/she wind down slowly with quiet activities as bedtime approached? Does the child routinely consume beverages containing caffeine or a high sugar content? Did he/she go to bed exceptionally tired or past the usual bedtime on the night of the attack? Were there any interpersonal problems or was anything at all bothering the child before going to bed? Were you at home or on vacation? Was the child sleeping in his/her usual bed? Did he/she get out of bed or just sit up? Did he/she actually walk or run around the room or even out of the room? What was the child's body language like during the attack?

Write down everything you observe. A sample log entry might be:

1/17/02: Last night, at my sister's house, Johnny had a very loud night terror attack fifteen minutes after going to sleep. He was sleeping in his cousin's bed at the time. He had not taken a nap during the day. He was sitting up in bed scream-ing and making choking noises for a couple of minutes and then fell right back to sleep. The next morning he remem-bered waking up and said it was because he felt like he couldn't breathe.

Over time you will begin to see patterns emerge after analyz-ing and combining many log entries. Every few months you should summarize your entries and findings. A sample summary might be:

Johnny began his night terrors at around age two. There was only screaming and no words. At first they were very frequent but eventually tapered off. Then at age four they started being frequent again. It happens about twice a week and lasts only about five minutes. Approximately 15 min-utes after going to bed we hear a loud scream. When we go into Johnny's room he is sitting up on the bed wildly waving his arms. He has usually kicked the blankets off onto the floor and sometimes falls on the floor himself. His eyes are wide open and he is sweating, crying, screaming, and mak-ing choking noises even though we know he's not choking on anything. His heart is beating very fast. He's in a panic. He does not wake up and doesn't respond to our questions. The attacks hardly ever occur on the nights when Johnny has napped during the day. The next morning, he sometimes remembers a little something about the attack and tells us that he felt like he couldn't breathe. Johnny has recently stopped drinking sodas containing caffeine, and we immedi-ately noticed fewer night terror attacks. During the summer, we spend every Wednesday at the beach. Johnny comes home more tired than usual and our log shows consistent night terror attacks on Wednesday nights. Last Saturday we stayed at Grandma's house. Johnny broke Grandma's lamp with a baseball and got punished. That night, while sleeping on Grandma's couch, he had an exceptionally long, loud,

and animated night terror attack. Come to think of it, he
seems to have a night terror attack every time he sleeps over
at my sister's house or we stay at a hotel.

The calm parent should observe and note the actions as well
as the words. Over time, this may give some hint as to exactly
what this "fear of the mundane" entails. Enough clues may be
given over time to enable the parent to address this fear or circumstance directly.

Diligent documentation will become more detailed and more
filled with patterns or conclusions over time. Additionally, your
calm, controlled understanding can only benefit the child. Thinking,
observant parents will almost definitely shorten the time it takes
for the Type A Night Terrors to resolve themselves. You might
also try casually talking to the child if he/she wakes up after an
attack, or on the morning following an episode, to see if he/she
remembers anything. Don't press the issue too strongly or for too
long as this will lead to apprehension. Just matter-of-factly ask if
the child remembers anything at all, or have him/her draw a rep-
resentation using colors. Children may go for months with no recall whatsoever and then begin to be able to remember faint
details. As Carlson and White reported after analyzing Dr. Fisher's
studies: "Through *careful* interviews, they determined that more
than 50 percent of the patients could recall some content when
closely questioned immediately after the event." (20, p.458) Very
careful interviews will result in a higher percentage of recall.
Write everything down in the log. *The Diagnostic and Statistical
Manual of Mental Disorders* states that "older children and adults
provide a more detailed recollection of fearful images associated
with [night] terrors than do younger children, who are more
likely to have complete amnesia." (3, p.585) If the child is verbal
and awakens immediately after the night terror, a couple of quick
questions while walking him/her back to bed may add up to a
recognizable picture if written down and analyzed over time.

It also wouldn't be a bad idea to allow the child to spend some
time around younger children. If Johnny's night terrors began

around age two, he might benefit by interaction with two-year-olds. Now that he's older, some valuable connections could be made in his mind. The older child may see that at the earlier age, children are more afraid of events they don't understand. Having the child spend time with younger children should be handled discreetly so that he/she does not lose self-esteem by getting the idea that you think he/she is a "baby." Rather, you should encourage the child to feel that he/she is helping you take care of the younger children. If handled properly, the child could thereby possibly gain some insight into his/her own fears by making waking connections with those "fears of the mundane" that he/she observes in the younger children.

In trying to make waking connections we are attempting to speed up the same process that the subconscious is trying to accomplish by dreaming. Dr. Hartmann contended that making connections is one of the primary functions of dreaming. He wrote: "We can make connections and thus become conscious of material, especially emotional material, that we were not aware of in our conscious, focused waking thoughts. Because dreams make connections more broadly and more loosely than waking thoughts, and since our emotional concerns guide these connections, dream material often leads quickly to emotional concerns that had been neglected or perhaps pushed away (repressed) in waking." (27, p.173) Besides this, attempting to help a child in this way and in this environment is actually therapeutic. You would be providing a comfortable, unthreatening environment in the hopes of facilitating some subconscious connections. As Hartmann again wrote: "Dreaming and therapy fill somewhat similar functions. In other words, making connections in a safe place may be an important and useful process." (27, p. 138)

Now you can begin to see why parents are usually the best experts on their child's condition. A brief doctor's visit once a month or so reveals very little of the above. And since practitioners may fail to ask the right questions, they may write very little specific information in their charts. Over time these sparse notes reveal few patterns. You, on the other hand, may hear or observe something unusual about the child's most recent night terror attack and think about it for some time, brainstorm with friends or your spouse, and actually come up with an insightful, helpful, and innovative understanding. Once consistent patterns begin to emerge in your notes and log, you'll find that innovative and insightful theoretical speculation is not very difficult at all. You will certainly make some interesting connections about the relationship between the child's activities of a given day and a later night terror attack. Making adjustments based on these connections should help to diminish the frequency of the child's night terror episodes. This in itself might turn a formerly disruptive, frequent Type A Night Terror problem into a very manageable intermittent concern. And there's always the possibility that you could figure out the details of the main causal mundane stress to which the child is overreacting during his or her night terror episodes. This could even result in a total resolution of the problem.

Drugs

Should drugs that mask night terrors be used until the condition is outgrown? It depends on the severity of the symptoms. If the child experiences no more than about three dozen moderate night terror episodes per year, I would hardly think that drug intervention is called for. If, on the other hand, these episodes are occurring almost every night, or the child has seriously injured him- or herself, then drugs might be an option. All the prior strategies, such as daily naps, sleeping in the same bed, winding down before bedtime, no caffeine, trying to figure out the main causal mundane stress, etc., should be tried before looking for someone to administer drugs. If the log reveals any improvement in the condition, then you may wish to keep trying the drug-free approach. Drugs should definitely be a last option. If the disruption of the household is too intense, episodes are too frequent, or the child often gets hurt during night terror attacks, then it may be time to seek drug intervention. Be sure to take your log with you to any professional you consult. If you do, the professional will give you more respect and will be less likely to prescribe incorrect medication or give inaccurate diagnoses (See the chapter on solutions to Type B Night Terrors for correct and incorrect medications).

The best source of help with this decision is a doctor who deals *exclusively* with sleep disorders and has extensive experience using different drugs in different dosages on many children of different sizes and ages. It may be difficult to locate such a professional through most insurance plans, but you should insist on it. Otherwise, the child will be sent to someone who may have no expertise in sleep disorders. When you first look for a professional, ask if he or she knows the difference between Type A and Type B Night Terrors. You may have to define the terms. Then listen carefully as to whether the professional values your insights. Choose one that does!

Even after a sleep disorder specialist is found, you, the parent, will still remain the best person to monitor the situation. Keep a log before beginning to administer the drugs and of course continue it afterwards. In this way the professional will be able to document the effect conclusively. If you and the doctor wish to cut down the dosage in six months, you will be able to tell from the log whether this is a good move or not. If the drugs are ineffective, or the dose is too low, the log will also reveal that. If there are any side effects, changes in mood, temperament, weight, eating habits, alertness, daytime drowsiness, etc., they should also be revealed by the log. Hopefully, drug intervention will not be a long-term strategy and the information gained from all your log entries will pay dividends before too long.

The following chapters will better your understanding of the far more serious Type B condition, making you more effective in helping a child resolve his/her less serious childhood Type A Night Terrors. Also, an understanding of the far more serious Type B Night Terror indicators will help to bolster your peace of mind as the years go on. If, as the child grows, you see that he/she displays none of the personality characteristics associated with

Type B Night Terrors, then you'll be even more certain that you've been dealing with the Type A variety. If, on the other hand, the child is in the minority and is really suffering from Type B Night Terrors, the next two chapters will help you to determine this with a higher degree of certainty.

As to Type A Night Terrors, you'll be surprised how much more smoothly things go when you can relax, observe, and carefully document the child's condition. The terrors will go away eventually. Even if resolution does not come until the child is in early adolescence, having at least one relaxed, supportive, understanding, calm, and loving parent/caregiver can only help the child to cope with this condition and minimize the impact of the night terrors on other areas of his/her life.

Chapter 6

Type B Night Terrors

What is important in investigating child trauma is to question the severity, depth, meanness, damage, and/or length of the caretaker's/perpetrator's behaviors. This is particularly acute at the preverbal and early life stages when a child relies on caretakers to provide a safe environment in which to explore the unknown. If that environment is not safe, the emotions of fear, tension, hurt, and frustration flood the mind, cloud thinking, slow and even prevent learning and growth.

Patterns of feeling, thinking, and behaving are formulated in these early years. This mostly unconscious process follows each individual into adulthood. The child has no way to counter the damage of abuse because he/she has no reality-checking experience. Lacking abstraction and critical reason, all children develop defense mechanisms which protect them from the bad feelings, thoughts, and behaviors of themselves and others. Such mechanisms as denial, avoidance, rationalization, etc., used to survive severe situations, may protect the child/adult for the moment but may be played out in the unconscious, resulting in sleep disturbances.

As already explained in depth, the difference between the two types of night terrors is stark. Type B Night Terrors are a much rarer, lifelong malady, now proven to be a persistent consequence of extreme trauma. They will not simply go away by themselves. A failure to recognize the enormous scope and multiple negative offshoots and ramifications of Type B Night Terrors has made this malady extremely difficult to comprehend, let alone treat. Like an iceberg, the great majority of the devastation this disorder causes is below the surface and therefore unseen. Nocturnal symptoms, the actual night terror attacks, are obvious to anyone. What goes totally undetected and unrecognized is the nonstop, ever-increasing destruction that Type B Night Terrors cause in every phase and area of the victim's life.

Along with sleep problems, secondary complications including health and interpersonal problems are also found among Type B Night Terror sufferers. These secondary complications, and societal ramifications have always added to the night terror victim's woes. During various epochs, night terrors were attributed to such causes as insanity, witchcraft, or demonic possession. Fortunately, today's societal ramifications are usually limited to cruel laughter, ridicule, demeaning judgments, and embarrassment. However, with reliable guidance and direction, most of the mystery surrounding this malady should dissipate. Type B Night Terrors, though stealthy and evasive, leave fingerprints and footprints everywhere. The condition can therefore be identified, tracked down, and subdued by carefully exposing and examining numerous telling details.

One of the many reasons that most professionals have little understanding of Type B Night Terrors is that they don't question the easily acquired details. They blindly trust the wrong sources in obtaining the patient's history, without giving very much thought to the veracity of the account. The facts say one thing, while the parents, the night terror sufferers, or others who come to the doctor's office and relate their stories for them say something else. Because of the generally accepted theory that night terrors are genetic, the professional hears exactly what he expects to hear from a parent or other caregiver who may have a personal motive for not telling the entire truth. (This is the same reason Munchausen by proxy syndrome went undetected for decades.) Abusive parents were able to put on a charming show and thereby deflect suspicion away from the fact that they themselves were the perpetrators of the abuse.

There is much more on phony abusers later, including the life-long propensity for Type B Night Terror sufferers to become involved with the same kinds of empty, dysfunctional, insincere, and dangerous people as those who abused them. Now that we know the true causes of Type B Night Terrors, this connection makes perfect sense. Children from alcoholic homes often end up in adult relationships with alcoholics. Battered children often end up in adult relationships with violent wife beaters or other types of batterers. These consistent patterns have been attributed to "going home syndrome" (duplicating the dysfunctional home one grew up in); resuming unfinished business from childhood; saving the abuser; associating turmoil with "love," since the two were synonymous in childhood; having become immune to or comfortable with extreme dysfunction; or simple emotional blindness. Children often have to become emotionally blind to the carnage in their homes in order to survive. It's a well-known fact that this childhood blindness oftentimes carries over into adulthood. Blindness to alcoholism or battering is easily understood. The extreme emotional blindness Type B Night Terror sufferers have to develop is multifaceted and complicated yet well documented, and once explained, relatively straightforward.

The door to the widespread acceptance and comprehension of the broad range of Type B Night Terror ramifications, manifestations, and offshoots has recently opened. We now know that if a human psyche is struck with extreme, intolerable force, the brain and nervous system are likely to suffer substantial damage, which will later manifest itself in the form of night terrors or other anxiety disorders.

A few years ago, The American Association for Marriage and Family Therapy published one of my articles in their *Family Therapy News*. It explained how extreme trauma causes radical changes that lead to the development of Type B Night Terrors. While there were no laboratory studies supporting this premise at the time of publication, today's science has proved my writings to be accurate—but only for traumatized children. I'm certain that the same negative biological mechanisms also occur in adults. Mood, anxiety, and sleep disorders are the result of extreme trauma in all the adult scenarios that I've documented. Therefore, I believe that the same chemical brain changes take place when an adult is subjected to extreme trauma. *Regardless of age, if a human being receives an extreme blow to the psyche (in one form or another), the resultant biological changes lay the groundwork for the development of Type B Night Terrors.* No matter which scenario is examined over the years, the results are the same. The following are some powerful examples:

- When Jewish human beings (both children and adults) suffered an extreme blow to the psyche (in the form of a Nazi concentration camp) they later developed Type B Night Terrors.
- When sea-going human beings suffered an extreme blow to the psyche (in the form of a horrific marine disaster) they later developed Type B Night Terrors.
- When human prisoners of war suffered an extreme blow to the psyche (in the form of torture in World War II, Korea, and Vietnam) they later developed Type B Night Terrors.
- When humans serving in Vietnam suffered an extreme blow to the psyche (in the form of witnessing and participating in nonstop death and carnage) they later developed Type B Night Terrors.
- When young human beings suffered an extreme blow to the psyche (in the form of the Chowchilla school bus kidnapping) they later developed Type B Night Terrors.
- When Dr. Marshall's patients suffered an extreme blow to the psyche (in the form of surgical complications, an electrocution, and an industrial accident) they later developed Type B Night Terrors.
- When the author of this book suffered an extreme blow to

the psyche (in the form of extreme infant and early childhood abuse) he later developed Type B Night Terrors.

The only thing that was different in each of these scenarios was the form the extreme blow to the psyche took. The fact that the "weapon" that struck the psyche was different in each of the examples appears to have confused many. Would anyone have failed to see the obvious if the "weapon" and the damage were physical? If literature documented clubs, large stones, and axes forcefully impacting human skulls, would anyone have trouble comprehending an association between the trauma and the result simply because the weapons differed? Like other researchers, M. Mahowald and G.W. Rosen may have overlooked clear-cut scenarios, such as the above, when they wrote: "There is little evidence that the majority of either children or adults experiencing [night] terrors have any significant underlying psychiatric disease or psychological problems. The most important underlying factor is a genetic predisposition." (29, p.31) Otherwise, the trauma connection would have been obvious to them.

The inverse of the above is also true. If an adult has been suffering from Type B Night Terrors for his/her entire life, then this specific manifestation of trauma-related brain damage is indisputable evidence of past extreme trauma. Decades after the fact, it may be impossible to locate or specifically identify the exact circumstances of the trauma that took place in infancy or early childhood. But just as the bleeding, cracked skull testifies to the fact that some form of physical trauma must have taken place, Type B Night Terrors testify to the indisputable fact that some form of psychic trauma must have taken place.

Personality Characteristics of Type B Sufferers

Certain personality characteristics are associated with Type B Night Terror sufferers. While careful researchers have documented these patterns for decades, they have been unable to explain them. However, the literature is overflowing with observations about personality characteristics that are consistently demonstrated by Type B Night Terror sufferers. The following are a few pertinent examples.

"J. Kales *et al.* (1980), in a study of 40 adults who suffered from night terrors, evaluated personality patterns of these adults and found that they exhibited 'an inhibition of outward expression of aggression.' " (5, pp.186-187)

"This MMPI [Minnesota Multiphasic Personality Inventory] code pattern indicated a clinical picture that was characterized by passivity." (30, p.402)

"(Night terror sufferer) J.B., a serious, intelligent young man, held a responsible job and was taking graduate level courses as well. There was a feeling about him of considerable energy, carefully controlled." (31, p.504)

"The sleepwalkers showed active, outwardly directed behavioral patterns whereas the night terror patients showed an inhibition of outward expressions or aggression and a predominance of anxiety." (13, p.1413) (Sleepwalkers are in a different category from night terror sufferers, even though night terror sufferers may sleepwalk.)

"The predominance of 2-7-4 and 2-7-8 (test result) elements suggested a high degree of inhibition of aggressiveness and of assertive and demanding expression of anger. The elevations on the scale 8-Sc did not seem to reflect schizophrenic or other overly psychotic disorders, but rather suggested self-direction of anger." (13, p.1415)

"From a clinical standpoint, all three patients showed an inhibition of outward expressions of aggression, intense fears of failure, and a strong tendency toward internalization of their emotions." (31, p.405)

"Persons subject to consistent episodes of night terrors inhibit outward expressions of aggression." (20, p.462)

"Certainly these are people who don't act out on their impulses while awake." (Dr. Scharf, on the Oprah Winfrey show, April 6, 1996)

And finally, even back in 1983, Dr. Ernest Hartmann was on the right track when he wrote: "Persons with a tendency to 'hold in' or control their feelings excessively are the persons most likely to develop night terrors." (31, p.505) However, the correct order of events is reversed. While it is true that some people have a tendency to become somewhat repressed in their feelings, the kind of severe repression associated with night terrors is not caused by that tendency. In other words, the sufferers are not emotionally repressed people who later develop night terrors. They develop the night terrors first, because of abuse and psychic trauma. After that, they acquire the severe habit of holding in, controlling, and repressing their feelings in ongoing encounters with their oppressors/abusers. The correct causal sequence is clearly discernible in the Auschwitz cases. The majority of the survivors were not people who had an abnormal or severe habit of holding in, controlling, and/or repressing their feelings before they were interned. Before WWII, the majority of them were most likely normal people. It was only after the horrific treatment at the hands of the Nazis that they developed night terrors, and subsequently acquired the extreme habit of holding in and controlling their feelings in all future encounters with their torturers in order to survive.

Consistent personality characteristics emerge almost universally among Type B Night Terror sufferers. These people are very passive, carefully controlling their every emotional reaction or expression, internalizing their feelings rather than letting them out or acting upon them; and, most important, they show an "inhibition of outward expressions of aggression." This means that adult night terror sufferers characteristically cannot raise their voices, react strongly, or in any way express anger at anybody. This excessive passivity is curious. It points to yet another inconsistency, an occurrence that would not make sense if the origins of night terrors were genetic. *Why would people suffering from a genetic condition consistently display the exact same personality traits?* Were these individuals also predisposed to be repressed, expressionless, carefully controlled, and inhibited?

It's fairly well established that eye color is passed on genetically. Yet, there is nothing consistent about the personality characteristics of blue-eyed people. You would certainly not be able to look at people with blue eyes and see the kinds of consistent personality patterns that are almost universally found among Type B Night Terror sufferers. People with blue eyes display about the same mix of personality traits as any other cross-section of society. There is no uniformity in their personality patterns.

This leads to the question, Why would the night terror literature consistently reveal that night terror sufferers possess very definite consistent personality traits? These very characteristics had been an extreme and obvious part of my own temperament as far back as I could remember. I was always described as smiling, good-natured, mellow, easy to get along with, agreeable, self-controlled, peaceful, and never angry. Relatives say I displayed these traits even before I entered school. Teachers routinely noticed this. I always knew inwardly, and now I am able to describe outwardly, exactly how I got that way. These personality patterns were certainly not inherited.

There is definitely one major environmental stimulus, and possibly several minor ones, pushing the individual in the direction of these personality traits. I'll start with the stimulus that has the most impact. In talking about the Nazi concentration camps, Bruno Bettelheim wrote, "In general, prisoners remembered the details and did not mind talking about them, but they did not like to talk about what they had felt and thought during the time of torture. The few who volunteered information made vague statements, which sounded like devious rationalizations, invented for the purpose of justifying that they had endured treatment injurious to their self-respect without trying to fight back. *The few who had tried to fight back could not be interviewed; they were dead.*" (32, p.230)

The Holocaust survivors learned the same passive, expressionless internalizing and anger-restraining behavior as other Type B Night Terror sufferers. Dr. Eitinger noted the same personality changes and traits as Bettelheim and others.

People who were subjected to the extreme psychic stress of the concentration camps displayed very similar personality traits. They had learned to be repressed. They displayed no dramatization when telling about this horror; verbally and in every other way, they were not acting on how they felt. They seemed incapable of expressing their true anger. The repression that Eitinger said was the only way to cope was not a normal kind of repression. It was total, abject. One had to become fully "emotionally inhibited" and devoid of all reaction in order to survive. This would have to take place dozens of times a day. Those who could achieve such repression might live, and those who couldn't would only have to react once and they would die. The extinguishing or total suppression of this part of the psyche had to be complete and had to cover all circumstances. Ninety-nine percent wasn't good enough. The one reaction out of a hundred would be the last.

At first the pain of holding all this in was excruciating. Then emotional numbness set in. After months of this, the repression was complete and the victims' capacity to react was altered for the rest of their lives. Existing literature documents this same repression in almost all Type B Night Terror victims, not just the survivors of the Holocaust. So, not only do all Type B sufferers exhibit the same extreme condition as the Auschwitz survivors (their night terrors), they typically exhibit the exact same personality characteristics that enabled the Auschwitz prisoners to survive. Again, this is not a coincidence.

Additionally, all sufferers develop an inordinate ability to tolerate pain. Long after writing about pain tolerance, I happened upon an interesting quote in the book *Rebuilding Shattered Lives* by Dr. James Chu. He wrote: "[In] persons who were extensively traumatized in childhood, the ability to ignore pain is also frequently observed." (34, p.31)

Psychic numbing, a defense mechanism, also contributes to the development of some of the characteristics discussed above. Dr. Hartmann wrote: "The symptoms of PTSD include not only nightmares and flashbacks about the traumatic event, but also avoidance of any situation or feeling associated with the trauma, and sometimes a general detachment or reduced responsiveness known as 'psychic numbing.' These patients have developed a different style of existence, involving walling off the trauma and avoiding anything that might remind them of it, avoiding emotional relationships that might bring up painful memories and in fact avoiding emotion generally." (27, pp.32, 33)

Changes in Perspective

Many Type B Night Terror sufferers are also reported to be cheerful and optimistic. Defensive emotional blindness in conjunction with mind-altering changes in perspective probably factor into this optimism. The emotional blindness is a given. You cannot continue to function while being tortured unless you can successfully shut off the parts of the psyche that register physical and emotional pain. Type B Night Terror sufferers elevate this blindness and shutdown process to an art form. Later on in life, as we shall see in subsequent chapters, this blindness and severely limited emotional capacity inevitably lead to further problems and turmoil.

From as far back as I can remember, I've always played games with my own outlook in the form of strategies and viewpoints that fostered optimism. I was very surprised to read accounts of Holocaust survivors who employed similar strategies. When you have no power or autonomy, then the only opportunity for action may be to empower yourself in your own mind. Where you are powerless and tormented you attempt to cope by creating your own scenario or setting. Eitinger wrote about Holocaust survivors who made a point of taking their paltry ration of bread and dividing it into three servings. He said: "[They retained] the ability to make some of their own decisions. If only the decision was about how to deal with their meager daily ration of bread or keep up personal hygiene, the decisive factor was always that they did not consider themselves completely passive. They did not lose their reasoning power, their ability to plan and to put their plans into action." (33, p.300)

These prisoners empowered themselves by making it possible to eat three meals a day. It was a game they were playing with themselves. But it factored into their outlook, perspective, self-respect, and ultimately their survival. Many of the concentration camp inmates who did not play these mental games with themselves assessed the hopeless reality of their situation, became despondent, and threw themselves against the electric fences or committed suicide in other ways. Dr. Eitinger described these soon-to-be dead prisoners. Their demeanor was marked by "indifference, dullness, and apathy . . . when all mental processes are retarded and normal reactions cease. Life ceased to interest the prisoners and they gave up hope." (12, p.473) These writings caught my attention because I remember playing many similar games with my own psyche. These games did nothing to change the situation, but they fostered optimism by creating the illusion of actually having some control over it. The painful, hopeless situation couldn't be changed, so in order to keep moving forward, one's perspective had to change.

I know that my own outlook was altered very early in life. As a child, I told people that I only felt like a tormented cripple when at home. Outside the home I was freer and more filled with joy than the normal kids. While, inarguably, the joy outside the home was an emotional delusion and an escape, the perspective gained contained some reality. In my choice of the word "cripple" I was comparing myself to several mentally retarded, wheelchair-bound children whom I knew very well. However, in contrast to my own situation, their struggle was full-time with no change in status regardless of changes in environment.

Also, the timely exposure to good, caring people outside the home definitely helped to change my outlook. Dr. Morrissette studied the long-term ramifications of child abuse and found that "availability of support" factored into "a healthier level of adjustment over time." (36, pp.82, 84) In other words, abused children who were fortunate enough to encounter people who took an interest, people who showed love, and people who listened fared better than those abused children who had no support. Good-hearted neighbors routinely comforted me. The mothers of my friends talked with me, fed me, and made me feel like part of their families. A loving aunt and uncle let me live out-of-state with them for several successive summers. A sixth-grade teacher, Thelma Singer, with the approval of her sister, the principal of the school, devoted a huge amount of time and energy to me. For a full year she worked ceaselessly at making a difference in my self-esteem, education, development, and outlook.

Of course, I still had night terrors; the biological damage had been done. But without the support of caring people, I do not believe that I could have kept moving forward effectively. Abused children without support oftentimes have their development slowed. In those cases, the dysfunction of their homes infects not only their emotional well-being but every part of their growth and lives.

Life also improved the older I got. My abuser feared exposure. So, when I developed verbal skills and contacts outside the home the abuse became less blatant. My increase in size and strength also diminished the level and impact of the abuse. This steady improvement probably resulted in increased optimism as I increased in age.

My optimism and improvement in life may have also been bolstered by an improvement in my friend-selecting process. Up until fifth grade I was always befriended by the school bully and the angry, volatile, violent, and dysfunctional kids that none of the "normal children" would tolerate. Other kids would not hang around these dysfunctional children for very long. Because of the anger I saw at home, the aggressiveness of these children didn't phase me. I was used to it.

By junior high school I stopped associating with angry kids. My friends were now severely depressed children. I didn't recognize that they were depressed at the time. I only saw that they were deep, intelligent, troubled, and quiet boys. Only years later, upon learning that three of my friends had committed suicide, did I recognize that their words and behaviors had been signs of fatal depression.

I had never entertained suicidal thoughts and attributed this to the perspective and emotional blindness developed during my up-bringing. Once outside of such an abusive home, what could possibly make me depressed and angry? I couldn't even recognize when I was under attack, let alone be bothered by it.

Recently, another of Carol Glod's findings caused some questions to run through my mind. She wrote: "The abused group displayed higher levels and percentages of nocturnal activity compared with both normal and depressed subjects. Children with PTSD but without depression slept much more poorly than those with PTSD and depression." (10, pp.1239, 1240) The children in her study were suffering from either sleep disruption or depression. It was one or the other. Is that part of the reason Type B Night Terror sufferers are typically not depressed but optimistic, active, and forward moving? Did my violent, emotion-filled night terror attacks act as some sort of emotional release or safety valve, and does the routine release of this emotion allay some kinds of depression?

Secondary Characteristics

In his study "Organic and Psychosomatic Aftereffects of Concentration Camp Imprisonment," Dr. Leo Eitinger found a universal consistency in both the physical and mental "deterioration" of those who had been "systematically tortured" by the Nazis. Besides correctly theorizing that "organic cerebral damage" was responsible for "sleep disturbances . . . anxiety . . . and *impaired memory* and *retention,*" Eitinger also documented the following: "Premature aging and *frequent illness* were general. Among diseases of the respiratory organs, *chronic bronchitis* was predominant, often combined with asthma, emphysema, bronchiectasis, and *chronic sinusitis. A lowered resistance to respiratory infec-*

tions was common. Psychiatric disorders appeared with greater frequency among those who were under the age of 25 at the time of arrest. The main symptoms were: *poor memory* and inability to concentrate. Anxiety was very clearly associated with *nightmares and sleep disturbances.* They had received no psychiatric treatment either, and their symptoms had to become chronic. We wish to emphasize again that the nightmares described by our patients were *always related to actual circumstances in the past* and that their contents were thus very real." (37, pp.109–111)

Eitinger clearly recognized all the symptoms because he had been in Auschwitz and had suffered from many of those after-effects himself. I recognized the veracity of his writings because chronic bronchitis, sinusitis, respiratory infections, and breathing allergies had ravaged and negatively impacted my life for decades. Constantly sneezing, coughing, struggling to breathe, pumped full of antihistamines, decongestants and antibiotics, and battling unabating bronchitis for four to eight months out of every year comprised my daily existence for decades. On top of this, Dr. Fisher and many other researchers have documented the link between sleep deprivation and increased night terror activity. The more tired you are, the deeper you sleep and the more likely you are to have a night terror episode. Fisher wrote: "One of the most striking and significant findings is that the night terror is linked to the presence of stage four sleep, its intensity closely correlated with the amount preceding its sudden onset." (14, p.93) Additionally, studies show that being sick during the day leads to more intense and frequent terror attacks at night. Kales wrote: "The initial suppression of stages 3 and 4 sleep with high fever may be followed by a rebound in the sleep stages, predisposing subjects to disorders of arousal from slow-wave sleep. Our contention is supported by Fisher and associates' suggestion that longer periods of stages 3 and 4 sleep preceding a night terror episode result in a more intense episode." (26, p.1215) So, continual health problems result in an increased incidence of night terror attacks of a more violent nature. Correspondingly, disrupted sleep and nighttime stress aggravate the already out of control respiratory ailments. It's a vicious cycle that will grow and feed on itself year after year for a lifetime if not checked. This cruel disorder is not satisfied with destroying its victims' sleep and psyche at night; it also destroys their physical health and well being during the day!

Fortunately, once I was able to make the connection between Dr. Eitinger's findings and my lifelong respiratory health problems, I had some direction. Realizing that lifelong Type B Night Terrors had caused a deterioration of my immune system and lowered my resistance to respiratory ailments, I began following some of the steps that kidney and other transplant patients take. They become very careful about exposure to germs, knowing that the simple cold that is only a minor inconvenience to a healthy individual can put them back in the hospital, or worse. I did the same things that transplant patients do: I washed my hands often. I would avoid anyone who was sick, even my own wife and children. As often as possible, I prepared my own food. I stopped playing indoor basketball during winter months because of the close proximity and contact with people who were beginning or ending a severe cold or flu. I wore a dust mask when around cats, weeds, or other things I knew I was allergic to.

I knew that every time I got a cold or severe sinus problems it evolved into bronchitis. I also knew that every time one of my children brought home a contagious disease from school they would get over it in a week or so. After I would contract it, the ailment would lead to severe respiratory problems and bronchitis that I would battle for the next two months or so.

At the same time that I was actively addressing my health issues, I was also beginning to get a handle on my past and present emotional life. My night terror symptoms were diminishing as my health was improving. I seemed to be dealing with both problems simultaneously. The vicious cycle of health problems by day and Type B terrors by night was being attacked on two fronts. The results were impressive.

I'm sure that the emotional breakthroughs and waking connections I was making were more responsible for my improved health than anything else. But it helped to know that a deteriorated immune system and a lowered resistance to respiratory ailments were also related to Type B Night Terrors. The awareness of secondary complications is a plus when dealing with any malady.

While many people do outgrow their respiratory problems and allergies by middle age, I doubt very much that that would have happened in my case without my having cured my night terrors. Rather than gradually improving as I got older, my respiratory problems and allergies had been worsening for decades.

I suggest that all Type B Night Terror victims pay special attention to their own physical health problems, especially if they are related to respiratory ailments. For many years psychiatrists dealt unsuccessfully with my night terror problem while allergists and other physicians dealt unsuccessfully with my upper respiratory problems. Had Dr. Leo Eitinger not diagnosed the connection and written about it decades ago, I would never have obtained relief from either problem. Type B Night Terror victims need to be especially aware of these secondary characteristics themselves, because it's almost guaranteed that the medical professionals attempting to treat either the physical or psychological manifestations of night terrors are not going to be aware of the connection between the two.

Impaired Memory and Retention

While the answers that Dr. Eitinger provided about the relationship between exposure to extreme trauma and the ultimate diminishing of memorization and retention skills did not lead to the kinds of life-altering solutions that his documentation on respiratory ailments had, this information was also invaluable. In regard to this observation, Eitinger was not alone. Dr. Paul Chodoff wrote that many of those he interviewed had "complaints of difficulty in remembering." (15, p.328) Almost all the Holocaust researchers who conducted personal interviews with the survivors noted this memory complaint frequently in their studies. But Dr. Eitinger's extensive interviews gave intricate details about memory impairment. He related the fact that many of these individuals, who had obtained advanced educational degrees before the war, now found their memorization and retention skills barely adequate to function in far less demanding intellectual settings. His writings provided extraordinary personal answers to questions that had deeply troubled me since seventh grade.

By seventh grade most subjects, including athletics, musical training, and especially math and science, had become easy for me. So, where was the connection to impaired memory? It was in Spanish! Since I did not have to study to do well in any of my other subjects, I devoted all my energy to that one subject. All this work did not keep me from failing Spanish that year. And yet with very little work, study, or effort I breezed through my other subjects. This made no sense. I questioned whether I was mentally gifted, as the ease and success in my other subjects suggested, or mentally retarded, as my exhaustively studious failure in Spanish suggested.

This paradox was repeated throughout my high school and college education. It never made sense to me, until I read what Dr. Eitinger had written about a prisoner who before the war had been a very sharp, college-educated woman and after the war developed memory problems along with suffering from "disturbed sleep and nightmares." Eitinger wrote: "This previously active, vital, and intelligent woman was *not able to learn Hebrew in spite of intense efforts* and in spite of the fact that she already learned quite a lot before the war." (11, p.171)

Of course! Learning a language is pure memory. In most other subjects one can study the morning of the test, retain the information for just a few hours, and do very well in the subject. Language is more cumulative.

The severely traumatized woman that Eitinger interviewed had not only developed sleep disturbances, she saw her once functional memory deteriorate dramatically. I had always known that my memory and retention skills were very inconsistent and horribly flawed. I marveled at the extraordinary memorization skills of most of the people I got to know well in my life, especially children. Did everyone I came to know have an almost photographic memory? Of course not! It only seemed that way to me because of my own deficiency in this area.

Almost a year after writing this chapter, I stumbled upon another of Dr. Hartmann's eloquent and precise writings in support of what life had shown me about impaired sleep and its effect on memory: "One large area of research deals with the possible role of REM sleep in learning and memory formation. REM deprivation interferes with learning, especially on relatively complex tasks [such as] *language learning.*" (27, pp.203, 204) Since effective REM sleep is essential to learning and memorizing a language and night terrors interfere with both REM and non-REM sleep, it's clear why Holocaust survivors suffering from night terrors found it virtually impossible—just as I did—to memorize a foreign language.

While poor memorization and retention skills are generally disadvantageous to normal functioning in daily life, evidence suggests that the limited ability to recall past trauma may be an essential defensive mechanism. In fact, the *Boston Globe* reported that a pill is being developed that will keep traumatic memories from becoming permanently engraved in the brain. Researchers at Boston University envision a time when rape, abuse, or terrorism victims may be given memory-suppressing drugs immediately after a traumatic event in order to prevent PTSD, flashbacks, and trauma-related sleep disruption currently prevalent among "3 to 8 percent of the population." There is suddenly widespread interest in this type of solution because "the terrorist attacks on Sept. 11 have made post-traumatic stress disorder an increasingly familiar diagnosis." (67, p.21)

Thermoregulation

Dr. Hartmann made another interesting observation. He wrote: "The third body of research led me to suggest that a function of REM sleep is the restoration or resensitization of norepinephrine-dependent systems in the forebrain. At the most basic levels such regulation involves the body's homeostatic mechanism, including homeothermy, the ability to maintain relatively constant body temperature despite variations of outside temperature. Carefully controlled studies on long-term REM deprivation show that this lack of heat control (thermoregulation) is what kills rats after several weeks of REM deprivation. I think it likely that the whole series of such control mechanisms may be similarly affected, but since the lack of heat regulation has the largest effect, it kills the animals before the other disturbances are very noticeable." (27, pp.204, 205)

Based upon the above information, it might or might not be possible that the continual sleep deprivation night terror victims routinely experience could lead to minor difficulties with homeostatic regulation (heat intolerance) as well. This would seem questionable, however, as I've never read about any such complaint in any of the night terror literature. I've included Dr. Hartmann's information just in case other night terror victims or sleep researchers reading this book have also noticed patterns of inappropriate heat intolerance in connection with night terrors or other sleep disorders.

Credit Where Credit Is Due

Long before the current increase of interest in this subject, I had already found most of the answers to my lifelong Type B Night Terror related questions, struggles, and difficulties through the earlier, valuable writings of Eitinger, Knapp and others. Their explanations and answers to my problems with sleep, learning, breathing, and other areas covered later in this book changed every single aspect of my life. It can loosely be stated that I was treated by a handful of conscientious practitioners who had died years before I ever stumbled across their work. These still unrecognized professional experts were so meticulous and thorough that they were actually able to help cure my Type B Night Terror symptoms posthumously.

Chapter 7

Clarifying the Diagnosis

If a child for any reason spent the beginning of his or her life in the care of anyone other than at least one truly loving parent, then determining whether that child is suffering from Type A or Type B Night Terrors is somewhat more complicated. Since the caregivers now dealing with the night terror problem cannot accurately trace the infant's history all the way back to the hospital bed, some time may be unaccounted for. With such children, the incidence of serious, trauma-related Type B Night Terrors increases dramatically compared to children who have spent most of their early years with loving caregivers.

In the book *High Risk* by Magid and McKelvy, the authors pointed out that: "Adopted children, or children who have spent some of their childhood in foster child care, account for a disproportionate number of unattached children." (38, p.148) Unfortunately, the same is true for children who suffer from Type B Night Terrors. The chance of a child encountering an adult who is angry and deranged enough to inflict the kind of extreme, torturous abuse that causes lifelong, traumatic Type B Night Terrors increases when the child has not been in the care of at least one loving parent for the greater part of his or her early childhood. Numerous negative scenarios then come into play. There are unwanted children, those of unmarried adults and/or teenagers, children born to drug addicts, children who were taken away from unfit parents before being put up for adoption, dysfunctional foster parents whose motives for taking in a child were impure, and the list goes on.

Incidentally, just because these children are adopted doesn't necessarily mean that the adoptive parents caused the problem. In the cases of unwanted children, unwed couples, and drug addicted parents, the abuse was probably perpetrated upon the child by the biological parents. The adoptive parents may be functional, loving, caring people who wanted the child but adopted the Type B Night Terror sufferer after the natural parent(s) abused him or her. Subsequently, the statistics showing a greater incidence of abuse among adopted children may sometimes be related to the circumstances that caused these children to be put up for adoption in the first place, rather than to the later care of adoptive parents.

Extreme, conscienceless brutality toward an infant, which is rare with those loving parents who want the child, becomes more likely with an infant's exposure to people who have no emotional connection to that infant, and possibly worse yet, no emotional connection to themselves. However, both strangers and biological parents can fall into this dysfunctional, emotionally unconnected category. In fact, when the perpetrator is the biological parent, stereotypical views often cloak the abuse and protect the dysfunctional perpetrator, as with Munchausen by proxy syndrome mothers.

These brutal biological parents are almost always highly dysfunctional people and usually live under interpersonal circumstances that are quite bizarre. If the parents are highly dysfunctional, and/or the child is unwanted, then extreme brutality can also be perpetrated by natural parents. Like strangers, these parents, too, can lack emotional connection or have a very weak emotional connection to the child.

It is important that there be a long enough period where the child is wanted and loved by a caregiver in order for complete bonding (emotional attachment) to take place, especially during the first year of a child's life. Unfortunately, it often becomes difficult to document what has actually taken place during the earliest formative years, particularly when the child has not been with the natural parents for a great part of that time or those parents happen to have been highly dysfunctional. However, aside from the issue of documentation, it needs to be emphasized that the key to an emotionally healthy beginning of life is being wanted and loved, whether it be by the natural parents, adoptive parents, or some other loving caregiver.

If you are a parent of an adopted child who suffers from night terrors, it is certainly painful to have to consider that the child may have come from a highly traumatic background. The easiest thing to do would be to bury your head in the sand and ignore all peripheral signs. But apathy isn't an option! The night terror war is being fought nightly in your home, and the casualties are your entire family.

While loving parents of wanted children who have been with their offspring from birth can be supremely confident that they are only dealing with temporary Type A Night Terrors, parents of unwanted children or those of adopted children may want to seriously consider the possibility of Type B Night Terrors. Unfortunately, unless you know for sure that your child had been abused before adoption, you may have to wait for the emergence of additional signs in adolescence before a reliable diagnosis can be made.

Adolescents comprise a gray area when it comes to diagnosis. Are they suffering from trauma-related Type B Night Terrors, or are they suffering from casual Type A Night Terrors that are just a little late in resolving themselves? By their teens the sufferers are old enough to help provide some clues. First, they can tell you about the actual visual content of the night terror itself. If closely questioned immediately after the attacks, they should be able to remember something. Persistence in attempting some recall can yield helpful information.

For years the literature has documented consistent themes that are commonly associated with night terror attacks. Fisher reported: "The major themes of night terrors were fear of being crushed, enclosed, abandoned, choking, dying, falling and fear of aggressive acts by others." (39, p.186)

The most universally reported theme is that of choking or not being able to breathe. However, the consistency of the visual content that night terror victims were reporting made little sense while the genesis of the condition was believed to be genetic. Remember that almost all the Holocaust researchers documented a definite link between the past experiences in the concentration camps and the content of the night terror "dream." It was repeatedly noted that the survivors were bolting out of their sleep screaming about things that had actually happened to them while imprisoned by the Nazis. Even the non-Holocaust researchers like Dr. Fisher found that the "mental content associated with the night terror episodes is often recurrent, sometimes linked to definite pre-existing traumatic experiences." (14, p.94)

And Dr. Terrence L. Riley wrote: "In adolescents the [night] terror is more typical of that seen in the adult, beginning very suddenly with a scream, usually followed by broken phrases that suggest concern of attack—'It's going to get me, I'm going to be crushed'—abandonment, aggression, or death (Fisher, Kahn, Edwards, et al., 1974)." (40, p.139) Susan Knapp observed something similar: "The sleeper appears to attempt to fight or flee. Stern (1951:302) referred to these episodes as 'one of the most striking manifestations of anxiety in human life.' " (5, p.180)

Not until covert Munchausen by proxy videotape discovered that the number one act perpetrated on infants by their own mothers was an attempt to suffocate the infant with either pillows or the mother's body did people start seeing the obvious. *Being suffocated or choked is the number one night terror recall, precisely because suffocating or choking infants is the number one act perpetrated by sick abusers.* Now the consistency found in night terror "dreams" makes perfect sense.

Carefully interview the adolescent night terror sufferer immediately after the episode and also the morning after the night terror attack. Carlson and White's findings, quoted earlier in the book, are supported throughout the reliable literature. In the majority of cases, careful and pointed timely interviews should result in some "dream" recall. Write down everything the child or adolescent says. Do not ask leading questions like "Were you choking?" Let them remember or not remember. But do note if the theme is consistently about experiencing aggression from others, being choked, or not being able to breathe.

Also, begin paying attention to whether or not the patient exhibits some of the personality characteristics of the Type B Night Terror sufferer. Preeminent among the personality patterns is "the inhibition of outward expressions of aggression." If he or she settles everything calmly, is overly passive, never raises his voice to any adult, has a lifelong pattern of trying to reason with angry, volatile people, and most important, rarely expresses anger toward any adult regardless of the circumstance, that patient fits the pattern.

Is the child or adolescent overly good-natured, mellow, or peaceful to an extreme? Is he or she often befriended by the bullies and angry kids whom other children shun? Is the child's behavior the exact opposite of what a depressed child would exhibit under most circumstances? If physically attacked by a peer, is he or she not able to muster up enough anger to react, defend him- or herself, or fight back? Any of these observations that apply should be carefully documented and considered. Many times it's the overly easygoing nature of these children and adolescents, and the fact that they rarely initiate or are involved in any trouble, that causes parents, teachers, and others to dismiss the possibility that there may be psychological aberrations associated with their sleep disturbances. People are more likely to suspect prior abuse or home dysfunction as the cause of sleep disturbances in the angry, volatile, troublesome child.

If, in addition to night terrors, the adolescent has had a history of upper respiratory, bronchial, asthmatic, acute sinus, or breathing-related allergy problems, that could also be telling. Memory problems might also be contributing signs. If the incidence of night terror attacks and the severity of the episodes get worse during adolescence, this may be another hint that you're dealing with

Type B Night Terrors. I suspect that the same mental and emotional growth and awareness that cause Type A Night Terrors to disappear at this time also cause some Type B cases to actually intensify and get worse.

While cumulatively these general guidelines may be revealing and helpful, there is an even better hope for night terror diagnosis on the horizon. Since the *JAMA* study was actually able to measure chemical brain changes in persons known to have been abused, the same test should soon be available in cases where abuse is a possibility. In the near future, young people suffering from night terrors will be able to be tested. Chemical analysis will make an absolute diagnosis as to whether the child or adolescent is suffering from Type A or Type B Night Terrors. Such testing will eliminate all guesswork and make the correct diagnosis possible long before the sufferer reaches late adolescence or adulthood.

But until then, if the night terrors continue into late adolescence, the parents may wish to consider the following words by Dr. Carol Glod: "The present study confirms clinical observation that sleep is impaired in abused children. . . . Thus, if a child presents with impaired sleep, *abuse* (particularly physical abuse) *should be considered* as part of the differential formulation. Likewise, when evaluating a child who has been abused, sleep should be carefully assessed for clinically significant impairments." (10, p.1243) Obviously, if night terrors persist into late adolescence, then the chance that they are temporary, casual Type A Night Terrors decreases dramatically. However, self-resolution does occasionally occur that late in life.

On the other hand, if you are an adult past your early twenties and you have suffered from night terrors since childhood, then time has made your diagnosis for you. You have a very serious condition, Type B Night Terrors. The more benign Type A terrors would have disappeared by your early twenties at the latest. You can pretty much assume the existence of some extreme past psychic trauma because you have symptoms similar to those of the survivors of Auschwitz, and you exhibit the same manifestations as the brain-damaged abuse victims in the *JAMA* study. Refusing to recognize this is about as realistic as a malaria sufferer denying he was ever bitten by a mosquito. The proof is in the pudding. Trauma-related anxiety disorders do not arise unless there was a trauma in the first place. If at all possible, try to determine what the trauma was. Investigate whether or not your past included orphanages or foster homes. However, do not spend too much time on such a search, which in many cases will prove fruitless. Instead, make some logical and not so bold assumptions, and then get busy trying to understand as much as you can about Type B Night Terrors. Some of the primary as well as secondary characteristics and complications have already been covered. Common interpersonal problems, broader ramifications, further offshoots, and solutions will be addressed later on in this book.

Chapter 8

Coping with Extreme Trauma

It may be that those suffering from anxiety disorders, sleep disturbances, PTSD, and night terrors are the lucky ones among the abused and probably represent only the tip of the iceberg. Most of the women in the *JAMA* study somehow continued to develop emotionally and bond with other human beings in spite of their childhood abuse; in many cases they have grown into mostly functional adults who must unfortunately deal with anxiety disorders, sleep disorders, PTSD, or night terrors. The fact that they continued moving forward ultimately made them available for the study decades after the abuse occurred. Others were not able to do this. It goes without saying that those who committed suicide or turned to a life of crime, violence, and jail, or who never developed into sane or functional enough adults, would not be candidates for study.

The majority of severely abused children might be very difficult to locate and study. If a child's emotional growth is stunted and bonding with another human being does not take place, then mounting evidence suggests that he/she will grow into a manipulative, dangerous, angry, conscienceless adult. The angry mother who severely abuses her own children behind closed doors is the domestic manifestation of an unbonded individual. The conscienceless hoodlum or gang member who laughs when taking the life of an innocent stranger is the local societal manifestation. And the angry, sadistic mass murderer is the extreme societal manifestation. Is it coincidence that these prototypes are now surfacing in the news with increasing frequency?

The recent rash of high-profile child abductions and/or murders in San Diego and Stanton, California, Texas, Utah, and elsewhere throughout our country calls urgent attention to the fact that the number of predatory deviants among us is even greater than previously thought. Few of these people would ever volunteer for a study, since most of them act out their psychological disorders in secret. However, their psychotic behavior itself already shows that they have a lack of empathy for others, which is a frequent consequence of not having had the opportunity during the crucial formative years of life to bond meaningfully with at least one other human being.

Ken Magid and Carole McKelvy, in their 1989 book, *High Risk, Children Without A Conscience*, made a thoroughly compelling and convincing case for the importance of bonding. They wrote: "The problem starts at the beginning of life, when the scales are tipped toward a future of trust and love, or one of mistrust and deep-seated rage. . . . Once again the culprit is . . . pathogenic parenting . . . that arouses unconscious resentment and anger which persists into adult life and ultimately finds expression in the mistreatment of those who are weaker. It is useful to remember . . . that each of us is apt to do to others as we have been done by." (38, pp.ix, 67)

However, a minority of those who were abused as children do not do as was done to them. They don't become like their oppressors. They don't identify with their aggressors. They do not develop into hard, conscienceless, angry, cruel, deceptive, insincere adult "rage-a-holics." The infant bonding theories of Magid and McKelvy offer a plausible explanation as to why the majority of the severely abused become abusive adults themselves. But for the minority that do not, there are choices and coping mechanisms that come into play when the victims are old enough to rationalize.

Rationalization was touched upon in the section on perspective. It alters the way the individual perceives his or her environment and struggles. But the next step in the rationalization process involves decisions about how to cope. The most expedient coping mechanisms appear to be the most detrimental to the long-term emotional well-being of the individual. Dr. Eitinger explained this when he wrote: "There is no doubt that identification with the aggressor did occur in some prisoners. Interviews prove that identifying with the aggressor, as far as it occurred, was a negative coping mechanism, leading to destruction of those involved and—in the few cases where they survived—to deep pathological changes in personality." (33, p. 298)

While Eitinger readily admitted that survival had more to do with chance than anything else, he did find that individuals who were interested in the well-being of their fellow prisoners retained some semblance of individuality and ultimately had a better chance of surviving as relatively integrated persons. He also noted that "former prisoners show a greater sensitivity toward fellow humans, a greater capacity for empathy, and a greater appreciation for the higher values of life." (12, p.480)

Eitinger indicated that those who became like their oppressors (those inmates who policed their peers or enforced Nazi discipline upon their fellow prisoners) forfeited their last ounce of integrity, individuality, and humanity. This resulted in only a short-term benefit. In the short run, these individuals were fed better and treated somewhat better than their fellow prisoners. But in becoming like their oppressors, they had imposed a death sentence upon themselves. They were probably going to die because of being emotionally unprepared for changes. And even if they survived physically, the "deep pathological changes" that allowed them to act like the Nazis destroyed them psychologically. Either way, they were in essence dead.

By contrast, those who maintained their humanity had a better chance of surviving physically and retaining their individuality. But they also developed Type B Night Terrors. It may have been the least damaging option available under the circumstances, because suicidal depression or becoming like your oppressor is rarely the healthiest long-term choice.

The Charles Mansons of this world, the Type B Night Terror sufferers, the future child abusers, and some types of severely depressed people all experienced extreme abuse at some time in the past. What is it that made one fuse blow instead of another? Why aren't they all Charles Mansons, all Type B Night Terror sufferers, all child abusers, or all severely depressed individuals? My mother endured extreme child abuse and turned into an extreme child abuser herself. Why didn't I go her route? I strongly suspect the answer has to do with the five months of initial love, care, and bonding with Rose Carino in the orphanage at the very beginning of my life.

Bonding, when used in psychological terms, means that the child has a deep-seated feeling of being wanted, loved, and valued by at least one other person. It is the basis of a sense of self-worth without which an individual will usually grow up not giving any value to him- or herself, thereby being incapable of giving any value to any other human being.

In writing about this bonding process, Magid and McKelvy talked about a four-stage cycle that is necessary during the first year of life in order for bonding and attachment to take place. After the fourth stage is successfully reached, ". . . a sense of trust develops. Basic trust is comprised of three distinct parts—trust of self, trust of others and trust of humanity." (38, p.74) Without this bonding and trust in infancy, these individuals might grow into abusive, conscienceless adults who have no regard for the pain they cause other human beings. Magid and McKelvy wrote: "Wherever these people go a wake of misery and fear usually follows. Unknowingly we may be creating a society in which more and more people without conscience victimize the innocent. These deviants run the gamut, from child molesters, to abusers, to crooked entrepreneurs . . . to murderers." (38, p.ix)

Chapter 9

The Abused and the Abusers

The well-camouflaged, secret abusers may be some of the most dangerous people in our society. Anyone can detect and avoid the raging lunatic shouting death threats at everyone who passes by. Such persons are deeply disturbed at their core and their behavior lets you know that they should be avoided. Many people in our society are just as deeply disturbed at the core as these individuals, but they have spent a lifetime polishing an almost impenetrable facade of normalcy. In speaking about the mass murderer Ted Bundy, Magid and McKelvy wrote: "Bundy, in fact, fabricated the public Ted: scholarly, bright, witty, handsome. He developed the air of cool self-assurance, the look women found irresistible. Bundy's critical challenge from his teen years on was to perfect and maintain a credible public persona, *his mask of sanity.* He was lacking in true adult emotions, so he had to put on the look of normalcy while inside his rage went unabated."(38, p.63)

The initial behavior of these people, the mask, does not betray the anger, darkness, deception, and extreme dysfunction that fills their hearts. While Barbara DeAngelis (*Are You the One for Me?*) certainly felt for those who were abused as children and destroyed emotionally, she meticulously detailed the signs of the abused who have turned into abusers in adulthood. These people bring the "misery and fear" that Magid and McKelvy spoke of into the lives of unsuspecting partners. DeAngelis wrote of these "rage-a-holics": "They were physically, verbally, or sexually abused as child[ren] and stored up this rage inside, letting it out . . . when they feel 'safe.' Repressed grief from childhood gets acted out as rage in adults." (41, pp.173, 174) These people are exploding time bombs that continually go off on those too blind to get out of the way. They are continually erupting volcanoes decimating the emotional landscape of any human being who stays in their path.

What does this have to do with Type B Night Terror victims? As long as night terrors were attributed to genetics there was no logical association between rage-a-holics and night terror sufferers. Nevertheless, some had noted another of those curious unexplained "coincidences." Night terror victims often marry rage-a-holics. In the past, this finding made little sense. But as with many things, now that we know the true causes of Type B Night Terrors, it makes perfect sense. DeAngelis wrote: "You might attract an angry partner [if] you had one or more angry parents as a child, and you have anger and love closely associated in your mind. If you grew up with a 'rage-a-holic' you may have an extremely high tolerance for angry behavior, since it was 'normal' in your household. Sadly, people who are physically or verbally abused as children often grow up to be battered spouses." (41, p.175)

If this reason for the attraction between these two types isn't already fatal, it gets worse. Night terror victims are emotionally inhibited people who cannot express anger. DeAngelis explained that: "You might attract an angry partner [if] you have *a difficult time expressing your own anger.* I believe that we often unconsciously attract our opposites as partners in order to heal the imbalances in our own personality. The man who is emotionally shut down may attract a highly emotional woman; the woman who can't express anger may attract a man who is overly angry. The emotions you suppress, your partner may express." (41, p.175) And the abusive partner not only feels safe enough to continually explode, but the fact that the night terror victim cannot express anger actually causes the abuser to increase his or her angry attacks. DeAngelis wrote: "When you repress or deny your angry emotions, your partner picks those up, and they augment his own stored-up anger." (41, p.175)

Besides continually and overtly acting out their anger, these abusers also possess an overly defensive mentality and are therefore equally proficient at expressing their anger covertly. The initial lower level signs of a rage-a-holic are seen in the skills of eliciting sympathy, playing the role of the helpless victim, and then using that presentation to turn vicious character assassination into an art form. DeAngelis wrote: "Victims spend their time complaining about what's wrong. [They are] experts at blaming others for the problems [and] see life as an adversarial situation. Victims express their anger covertly. They may make statements that don't sound angry or hostile, but indirectly communicate their hostility while still allowing them to maintain the appearance that they're not angry." (41, p.180)

Females who are sympathy-seeking, overly defensive abusers play the role much more convincingly than men do because women are more easily believed to be sensitive, caring, vulnerable people. This is how the Munchausen by proxy syndrome mothers remained above suspicion for so long and why they were also able to convince doctors to abuse their children for them. Dr. Laura Schlessinger called these types of female abusive partners "damsels in distress." Schlessinger wrote: "Damsels in distress don't really want your help. Perhaps they want you to be their life or to give them a life and take responsibility for them so they don't have to exert effort to fix themselves. And so that you can be the one to blame when they just don't 'feel' better. And damsels in perpetual distress are usually wicked witches in disguise. Don't believe me? Well, just cross or disagree [with] or disappoint one—poof! Instant transformation." (42, pp.7, 23) These damsels may also be proficient at flattering, beguiling, and seducing male targets with their tantalizing but emotionally dead sexuality. Magid and McKelvy reported that these dysfunctional women "use sex as a primary technique of manipulation." (38, p.64)

Angry, aggressive men are not as prone to disguise their dysfunction because in many quarters of our society such behavior brings praise and admiration. The toughest boy in the school has both male and female admirers. The boy who channels all that anger and aggression into boxing or football may be praised for his athletic prowess and intense drive. He may be the envy of his male peers and the recipient of great attention from females. At the very least, most people will leave the angry male bully alone. Angry, aggressive women are not admired by their peers. Most girls exclude them. They're called bitches behind their backs. They are usually ostracized and verbally berated in secret or in the open by most girls their own age. These dysfunctional girls get an opportunity to practice their non-angry act, their mask of sanity, through simply trying to fit in with other girls, thereby allowing them to have a less painful school experience. Women are much better at seeing through other women than men are. So these women spend years practicing their deceptive art with an extremely critical and perceptive audience: other women. After years of such practice, they are very effective when throwing the same meticulously rehearsed pitches at sexually interested boys and men. Depending on the woman's physical appearance, numerous men may be willing to disregard their gut feelings and the glimpses of anger they've seen, and go on to date or even marry her.

Both male and female abused children who grow into manipulative, abusive spouses wreak destruction on the lives of their mates because these abusers have no business being in a marriage in the first place. In writing about these phony, detached individuals, Magid and McKelvy stated that: "[They] can forget about having any stable, long-lasting, intimate relationships, such as a marriage. [They] are incapable of forming lasting relationships, never becoming truly intimate and open with others. The manipulator appears to be helpful, even intriguing or seductive, but is covertly hostile, domineering, or at best neutral in interaction with another, whom he or she considers an object. This object is perceived as an aggressor, competitor, or instrument to be used. [They] cheat on their mates [and] carry diseases that they don't disclose." (38, pp.67, 10, 20, 307)

If the Type B Night Terror victim unwittingly follows his or her programming, then the person such a victim attracts and marries will likely be an angry rage-a-holic. The manipulative spouse will be continually acting out his or her lifelong rage on the emotionally blind night terror victim, who is unable to get angry or react. The victim might be trying to conduct a marriage, unaware that he or she is merely an object and the target of a sick, hostile soldier in an undeclared war. Sexual infidelity and promiscuity will be commonplace with such spouses, and their skill at self-delusion, character assassination, and playing the role of victim will allow them to self-justify all past, present, and future unwarranted anger and infidelity. As if the horrendous childhood, the lifelong history of Type B Night Terror attacks, the sleep deprivation, and the upper respiratory problems associated with this condition weren't enough, the night terror victim's marital life also becomes a living hell.

The sleep deprivation and continual health problems also add substantially to the victim's intellectual and emotional blindness and the likelihood of ending up in an abusive marriage. How can this person make sense of anything in the middle of all this turmoil? Simply surviving and coping with all of this is a full-time occupation for the Type B Night Terror victim. Not surprisingly, the lack of time to sort life out may also contribute to increased night terror activity. Sleep, a break from the conscious, may be one of the few opportunities for the victim to be unencumbered enough to even attempt to do the necessary sorting out. Dr. Hartmann wrote: "Indeed, at present many of us have opportunities to do some of this connecting while awake. Some of us have the luxury of a certain amount of leisure time. We can sit back, relax, work on problems. Our ancestors did not have much leisure time or time in a safe place to integrate traumas. Only [their] dreams gave [them] a chance to do this." (27, p.209)

Night terror victims are too involved in the war that is their daily lives to make any connections while awake. Their oblivious emotional state is also a roadblock to making waking connections. They have no mental leisure time; their minds are working full-time on survival. The only time left to attempt to integrate trauma is in the deepest stages of sleep. These victims are completely inept at making any sense of their waking emotional lives, much less making healthy and fulfilling relationship choices.

Most of the Type B Night Terror victims seeking treatment are probably involved in dysfunctional relationships. Why? As will be discussed in depth later, Dr. Leo Eitinger found that those suffering from trauma-related night terrors had decreased symptoms and episodes when they happened into peaceful, loving, and functional marriages. It can therefore be deduced that those who had an increase in night terror activity after marriage might be in dysfunctional marriages.

In the number of informal interviews I have conducted with night terror victims, many told of an unexplained dormant stage where night terror activity diminished. This was usually in early adulthood. I used to attribute this to the fact that at this age many victims went away to college, where they found atmospheres that were far more peaceful than at home. But then, why did the condition return with a vengeance somewhat later in life?

Most Type B Night Terror victims seek help only after their problem becomes intolerable after marriage. Is it because a mate is now being disturbed at night along with the sufferer? Or, as I now believe, did the mate contribute to a substantial increase in the amount of stress and turmoil in the night terror victim's life and thereby facilitate a new explosion of night terror activity? That would place the dormant stage squarely in between the time when the night terror victim left a parent's dysfunctional, stress-filled home and the time when the victim made the wrong choice in marriage and established his or her own dysfunctional, stress-filled home.

The likelihood that Type B Night Terror sufferers will end up in marriages to abusers increases even more because the abusers are the ones doing the seeking out. It's an advanced, logical progression of the same pattern that occurred in childhood. I didn't go looking for the angry, cruel bullies to befriend when I was a child; they found me. And for them, it wasn't so much a search as it was a process of elimination. The normal kids would simply not hang around with disturbed children for very long. The normal kids had a very low tolerance for anger, violence, unwarranted rage, and abuse. Magid and McKelvy asked: "What normal child would want to be friends for a long period of time when faced with a manipulative, self-destructive, and cruel 'friend'?" (38, pp. 90, 91) No normal child would. However, the child who was so severely abused that brain damage resulted, who leaps out of his or her sleep screaming at night, who represses all negative thoughts about anyone and has become totally oblivious to mistreatment by others, will tolerate a dysfunctional "friend." The dysfunctional develop an ability to spot children who are receptive to being manipulated and mistreated. This skill gets refined and perfected as these cruel children grow into adult rage-a-holics.

In referring to these skillful adults, Magid and McKelvy wrote: "They are generally not perceived as bad or evil. More often, they are charming and engaging. [They have] extrasensory perception about others and the ability to pick out personal vulnerabilities with uncanny accuracy." (38, pp. 11, 12) "[They] are capable of planning . . . and waiting for the 'right' victim or circumstance." (38, p.103) These abusive partners have found that relatively normal people are able to detect their insincerity and hostility and therefore get away from them. The abusers develop the ability to spot those who can be easily manipulated and who will tolerate their dysfunction and abuse. They immediately recognize and avoid those who are like them, and therefore will usually not end up in partnerships with their fellow abusers. Also, since this kind of dysfunction runs in families, female abusers have usually been able to learn what kind of males to avoid: men who are just like their abusive brothers or fathers. And male abusers have usually been able to spot what kind of women to avoid: women who are just like their abusive sisters or mothers.

The abusers seek out those who will tolerate abuse. Magid and McKelvy wrote: "Such manipulators often target church members and other individuals known for their generosity and naivete. Often the kind-hearted gestures are repaid with fraud and betrayal." (38, p.45) Thus, this constitutes another of the factors that increases the almost magnetic attraction. After spending a lifetime learning how to elicit sympathy and to pass themselves off as helpless, downtrodden victims, abusers actually target and seek out kind-hearted individuals, who because of their own legitimate past suffering are eager to help and trust the abusive wolf in sheep's clothing.

Furthermore, like many individuals who suffered early childhood abuse, Type B Night Terror sufferers are extremely vulnerable to dysfunctional abusers who are actively searching for someone they can sadistically exploit. Dr. Chu explained that persons who were abused in childhood are "intensely vulnerable to subsequent revictimization" and are easy prey for "predators who often search out those they can exploit." (34, p.107)

All of the above amounts to a classic case of overkill. Even the psychiatric professional is no match for the deceptive behaviors of these manipulative abusers. Dr. M. Scott Peck wrote that: "We see the smile that hides the hatred, the smooth and oily manner that masks the fury, the velvet glove that covers the fist. The disguise is usually impenetrable." (2, p.76) Magid and McKelvy concurred with Peck when they wrote that: "Psychiatrists are often helplessly manipulated." (38, p.22)

The emotionally unresponsive Type B Night Terror sufferer has absolutely no chance of seeing through an act that even trained professionals are unable to detect because of yet another factor, the well-documented defense mechanism of "psychic numbing" (mentioned in chapter 6). When an individual is subjected to a trauma that is beyond his or her capacity to endure, an emotional self-anesthesia mechanism often comes into play which dulls normal sensitivities and allows one to survive circumstances that would otherwise be intolerable. The Holocaust literature contains a great deal of information about "psychic numbing." This natural capacity to virtually stop one from feeling emotional pain ultimately kept those who survived the concentration camps from completely falling apart in the face of unending, nonstop horror.

This ongoing self-anesthesia is also the dominant defensive mechanism of all Type B Night Terror sufferers. It is the very thing that allowed them to survive childhood and also prevented them from turning into abusers themselves. Ironically, this past advantage becomes a present detriment. It's one of the primary factors that make Type B Night Terror sufferers such easy prey for those abusers who have targeted them, and who are on a mission to marry a punching bag so they can finally act out all their pent-up anger, rage, and hate on someone who is incapable of fighting back.

Relationship Problems of Night Terror Sufferers

In evaluating their Type B Night Terror patients, few professionals have paid close attention to the sufferer's adult relationships. But again, Dr. Leo Eitinger was keenly aware decades ago of the elusive connection between a night terror victim's traumatic past and his or her subsequent relationships. Back in 1972 he wrote: "The few whom this extermination apparatus had not managed to crush completely . . . were . . . absolutely without any form of anchorage in the world. This lack of anchorage, by the way, is very clearly illustrated by the numerous reports of marriages which often have only taken place because the partner chosen had an extremely peripheric connection with the survivor's earlier life, for example, he or she had known the 'father' or 'came from the same places as the parents.' This choice of partner, which was so often hasty and injudicious, led to later secondary complications." (11, pp.188, 189) In other words, victims will go on to make relationship choices that are completely arbitrary and haphazard, leading to the high probability that they will end up in an extremely dysfunctional marriage.

Dr. Eitinger also noticed the opposite happening in the many cases in which Holocaust survivors married fellow Holocaust survivors and both people shared strong Jewish family roots. Many were lucky enough to find themselves in marriages that were built upon secure social and interpersonal conditions. This group had less frequent night terror attacks. Eitinger concluded that the "creation of [interpersonal] bonds is essential for recovery from catastrophic stress." (43, p.171)

Wilise Webb made a similar observation. She wrote: "Recent attention to the relationship between highly stressful life events and nightmares has been very revealing. One researcher, Peretz Lavie, has reported that survivors from the Holocaust, who had made good adjustments, had less dream recall and disturbed dreams than those who had made less adequate adjustments." (7, p.101) Good adjustments after trauma, especially interpersonal adjustments and decisions, tend to positively influence the severity or frequency of night terror attacks, while bad interpersonal adjustments and decisions have a negative impact. There is no doubt about the accuracy of these observations.

The stress of the dysfunctional marriage is not the cause of Type B Night Terrors. Extreme psychic trauma is the cause of Type B Night Terrors. However, "hasty and injudicious" emotional and relationship decisions will lead to what Dr. Eitinger correctly termed, "secondary complications."

This becomes another of those vicious cycles. The typical adult night terror sufferer is prone to make arbitrary and unwise relationship decisions because the past severe trauma decimated, crushed, or repressed the parts of the psyche that are needed to make sense of his or her emotional life. Then, because the night terror is merely crouching below the surface of the subconscious, the added stress of the dysfunctional marriage is sufficient to aid in bringing the night terror episodes to the surface.

Let's not forget Dr. Fisher's experiment in which a bell that was set off during stage four sleep sparked artificial night terror episodes that were as intense as an unsolicited attack. If a bell was enough of a stimulus to bring night terrors to the surface, will the stimulus of living in marital turmoil be enough to do the same thing? Of course!

Just about the time that I was researching and documenting some of this information, Oprah Winfrey devoted a show to the subject of night terrors. Of particular interest to me were a night terror sufferer named Daniel and his wife Kathy. This mellow, seemingly sedated man sat there in a daze as his wife told about his night terror episodes. When in the throes of the night terror episode, Daniel's calm demeanor completely changed. He lashed out at Kathy with cruel and degrading words. As Kathy tearfully told her story, most of the audience empathized with her. Not only had she been awakened nightly but, during his night terror attacks, Daniel had screamed at her: "Wake up, wake up! I want to talk to you. I want you to die! You're a completely worthless person—you're wasting the air you breathe! I hate you! I want you to die! Why are you here?"

As has been discussed earlier in this book, are such words as those shouted by Daniel during his night terror attacks actually an expression of his true emotional feelings? This question was very interesting to me because shortly before viewing the program I had already concluded and written that: *"When the night terror victim is awake, his true emotional life is asleep. When the night terror victim is asleep, his true emotional life is awake."* (53, p.28) It is now becoming more and more evident that this is true, as confirmed by a variety of studies by reliable sources.

The wife (Kathy) then told of one of Daniel's more bizarre night terror attacks. He had awakened her one night with a knife to his throat, saying that he was going to slit his own throat and that when he woke up he would then think that she had done it and would slit her throat. It immediately dawned on me that even this man's night terrors were repressed. He would have to slit his own throat first and blame it on his wife in order to feel justified to slit her throat. Oprah Winfrey interjected, "Maybe he really thinks that about her. Is that his subconscious coming out here and saying all that?"

Was Kathy part of the reason for his latent explosion of night terrors? Like most other Type B Night Terror sufferers, was Daniel unable to even recognize an ongoing abusive situation, let alone react to it while awake? This seemingly catatonic man was obviously severely repressed. So, during his night terror attacks, was he releasing all his past and present repressed emotions, and were they being directed at the *appropriate target*? Was his subconscious coming out with what he really felt about his wife?

One of the medical experts on the show answered Oprah's question by saying: "Part of the brain is awake and part of the brain is asleep; beyond that we don't know—something about the emotional state as you fall asleep; we don't understand that." Then the expert made the following pertinent observation: *"Certainly these are people who don't act out on their impulses while awake."*

Daniel responded to all this by saying, "I love my whole family." He appeared somewhat oblivious while awake and suffered from chronic night terrors at night. But other than that, he seemed normal and was functional in most areas of his life. I suspect that the part of the brain that gets damaged and causes Type B Night Terrors also acts as a fuse. And although the fuse blows out, it leaves the rest of the person relatively functional and intact. One of the perplexing things to professionals is how otherwise normal many night terror victims are.

Back in 1983, Ernest Hartmann wrote, "There was no trace of psychosis or of depression, and no clear DMS-III diagnosis could be made, except for night terrors. It is striking to me that the two extreme cases discussed here [patients P.H. and J.B.] show so little psychological abnormality." (31, p.504)

While Type B Night Terror victims appear functional on the

surface, a deeper look reveals that their emotional lives are horribly flawed. Since night terror victims do not react, are oblivious to attack, and make "hasty and injudicious" emotional and relationship decisions, what else would you expect? As discussed earlier, they can get along with vicious, angry people that no one else can tolerate. For that reason, night terror victims are often chosen by people that no one else can stand to be around. They may spend their entire lives attracting, befriending, and even marrying the hostile, selfish people with whom no one else could possibly get along, people who have been looking for someone upon whom to vent their frustrations for their entire lives. In the night terror victim they find a perfect partner for themselves, someone who will let them explode at will and vent anger without any fear of repercussions. The angry persons now have the opportunity to pour out all their lifelong pain. They keep on pressing the attack, waiting to be stopped by some kind of reaction. No reaction will be forthcoming except at night. If it weren't for the night terror victim waking up the hostile partner at night there would never be any consequences for their unwarranted rage.

The lives of night terror victims become overloaded with stress that is predominantly from the home. They are unaware of being dragged to their emotional death, but their subconscious expresses outrage at night in the form of night terrors. So, Oprah's question turned out to be profound. Did she hit the nail right on the head? Was it really Daniel's subconscious coming out and saying all those negative things to Kathy during his night terror attacks? Does he really think that about her? I cannot answer these questions conclusively having only observed these two people on television. However, in my own case, in the cases of Holocaust survivors, and in many other cases throughout the reliable night terror literature, the words and actions during night terror attacks were very often directed at the appropriate target. The sleeping words of the night terror victim more accurately reflected the truth about the current emotional life and circumstances of the sufferer than his or her waking words. If the night terror victim is oblivious and repressed, and if the spouse is an angry pretender, a consummately proficient manipulator and liar, then the night terror attack itself and especially the words expressed might be the most reliable and informative witnesses. What was said should certainly be noted and carefully scrutinized. It may be pointing directly at the greatest source of unrecognized and unrelenting stress currently in the night terror victim's life.

Chapter 10

Two Contrasting Marital Case Studies

A few years ago I was fortunate enough to run across two men with sleep problems. One of them was not sleeping well because of stress and nighttime anxiety attacks, while the other was suffering from Type B Night Terrors. What caught my attention right away was that although the two men were unrelated by blood, they had married a pair of sisters from an extremely dysfunctional home. The nighttime anxiety attack sufferer, while looking for help and answers, was verbally guarded and evasive. On the other hand, the night terror sufferer, Joe, was both honest and forthcoming about everything he was able to perceive. Many of the things I had read about or concluded regarding the marriages of night terror victims came into much sharper focus after getting to know the details of Joe's marriage and especially about his wife.

Joe had suffered from night terrors his entire life. He had grown up in an extremely abusive home and still could remember many of the details about his torturous childhood. But, what made him so fascinating to me were his present circumstances.

Joe was seeing a competent, careful-listening therapist. He lent me a copy of his personal diary, which contained a great deal of information about himself, his therapy, and his wife. As he described both his upbringing and his marriage, it became clear to me that his wife exhibited many of the same extreme personality characteristics and aberrant behaviors that his parents had displayed as he was growing up. Was this simply coincidence, or was Joe's life an example of "going home syndrome"? In reference to this syndrome, Dr. Barbara DeAngelis wrote: "If love = home, and home = chaos, then love = chaos. Your unconscious mind will seek to complete its unfinished emotional business from childhood by getting you to 'choose' people who will help you re-create your childhood dramas." (41, p.54)

Although I had read extensively about relationships and had sought answers from therapists about my own interpersonal life, I was absolutely lost in making any sense out of Joe's situation. No self-help book covered anyone as pathologically unbalanced as Joe's wife. Most therapists Joe had seen were unable to make sense out of his wife either.

Joe had been married to Lucy for over ten years before extreme circumstances caused her to speak the very first meaningful words of truth she had ever spoken to Joe. It was only after these first significant truths were revealed that Joe and an astute therapist were able to accurately decipher the events of the prior decade. The monumental breakthrough came after Joe had decided to end the marriage. Joe had stayed together with Lucy in spite of her behavior and actions. She would routinely explode with anger over anything and then deal with it by calling up an old boyfriend and going out and having sex with him. In this way, she would "get even" with Joe.

Joe couldn't do or say anything right. Lucy was filled with life-long pain and took every opportunity to let it out. On top of this, any kind of communication only made matters worse. Lucy never had any interest in conflict resolution. She was simply listening for one word out of Joe's mouth that she could explode over and use as an excuse for further rage and extramarital sex.

Joe learned to deal with Lucy's overly defensive anger by being very careful about doing or saying anything that could in any

way be construed as an attack. However, he could never understand why the apparently normal, loving things he would do, or
the innocent words he would say, led to violent explosions that
sometimes lasted for weeks or months at a time. Needless to say,
Joe had constant night terrors during his marriage, and *Lucy was
always the focus of his anger and words during these episodes.*

Few people, professional or otherwise, could accurately relate
to Joe's situation. However, he was able to find some comfort and
answers by talking to his brother-in-law. It turned out that Lucy's
sister was as dangerous and explosive as Lucy. Joe's brother-in-
law told him about two recent events. The brother-in-law had
been thrown to the floor by Lucy's sister and then repeatedly
punched and kicked. He almost had his head split open when she
just missed striking him with a heavy object. What had precipi-
tated this rage was an argument over the kitchen mess he made
while making a sandwich. A week later he had to wrestle his
portable TV out of her hands in another episode. She was trying
to throw all his possessions out the window after blowing up because he had been snacking while she was making dinner. Lucy's
sister ended up in the hospital. She'd been badly cut after her arm
crashed through the window as Joe's brother-in-law was wrestling
the TV away from her. Numerous stitches were required to repair
the lacerations in her arm. Joe's brother-in-law ended the marriage shortly after that. He had had enough of the violence. Not
surprisingly, his nighttime anxiety attacks also stopped.

While both Lucy and her sister had experienced abuse in
childhood, Lucy usually released her resulting anger secretly and
in devious ways, while her sister habitually released her anger
with violence. Only on occasion would Lucy get violent. It was
after one such incident that Joe was ready to end his own marriage. Lucy had been calmly talking about an old boyfriend. Joe
mistakenly asked if that old boyfriend and another old boyfriend
he knew about had ever met each other. Lucy flew into a violent
extended attack like the ones Joe's brother-in-law had repeatedly
experienced. She was mad enough to kill! Joe and Lucy immedi-

ately separated. This intense display of unwarranted rage and violence was the last straw for Joe. Lucy moved back in with her dysfunctional parents and hostile siblings.

After a few weeks of interaction with her family, Lucy had become severely depressed and was even contemplating suicide. In desperation, she reluctantly began revealing information about her continual infidelity, deceptions and secrets. This eventually led to revelations about her earlier traumatic experiences. Lucy had been repeatedly sexually abused in childhood, scared by her violent, drunken father, raped and beaten as a teenager, and continually sexually used and exploited in early adulthood. Her life was dotted with abortions, underhanded deceptions, secrets, and nonstop ever-growing lies.

The explanation for Lucy's violent attack finally surfaced after Joe's innocent question about whether her two boyfriends knew each other. Some fifteen years earlier, she had stopped dating a man named Larry in order to date another, Hal. She then became angry with Hal and arranged to meet her married boss at a hotel; later, she claimed that he (the boss) had beaten and raped her, causing her to become pregnant. Lucy then returned to dating Larry and pretended for a month to be in love with him. She was planning to blame her rape-induced pregnancy on him, which she proceeded to do. After Larry paid for her abortion, Lucy exploded on him for "causing her so much pain by getting her pregnant and forcing her to have an abortion." She then went back to dating Hal, never told anyone about this scam, and tried to sweep the entire episode under the rug of her own consciousness. And there this painful secret remained until Joe accidentally lifted up the rug by innocently asking if these two boyfriends had ever met.

Most of Lucy's angry explosions had little to do with the present and even less to do with Joe. In fact, the majority of the aberrant behaviors she exhibited in her marriage were due to reenacting the past, or re-experiencing the latent discomfort associated with the momentary acknowledgment or remembrance of events from her thoroughly dysfunctional deceptive life.

For the most part, Joe had been oblivious to the significance of Lucy's continual animosity. Many Type B Night Terror sufferers *do not recognize their enemies*. After spending an entire childhood in the company of caretakers who hated them, *there is nothing unusual to them about being in close association with their worst enemies. In fact, trying to be intimate with someone who hates you is almost normal for a Type B Night Terror sufferer.*

Magid and McKelvy wrote something that is also applicable to Lucy. "Like someone on the outside looking in, they see another [person] who is happy, doing well. They think if they take what that [person] has they will have that happy feeling. They actually think that they can rip off happiness. It is impulsive, like a craving." (38, p.86) The Lucys of the world think that by lying and cheating their way into the lives of a person who is happy, somehow the happiness will rub off and they themselves will become happy. Of course, this doesn't work. So they blame their partner for the fact that they are still unhappy.

Lucy demanded that Joe make her happy, that he affirm her continually, and that he love her unconditionally. This was in spite of the fact she herself contributed nothing toward achieving these ends. She saw no association between her motives, behaviors, and actions and the desire we all have to be happy, appreciated, and loved.

Dr. Peck realized that people like Lucy never experienced or completed the phase of childhood where conditional love and a comprehension of good and evil take place. In speaking about one of his own patients, he said: "[Charlene demanded] that I love her regardless of how she behaved—that I affirm her . . . sickness and all." (2, pp.161, 181) He explained that Charlene understood enough about her life, her secrets, and herself to legitimately fear that she was unlovable and incapable of attaining affirmation by honest means. Furthermore, she took no responsibility for modifying her behaviors and attitudes, as normal adults do in order to help make themselves more lovable.

Lucy had also made some very bad, far-reaching decisions a long time ago. She was no longer going to be lied to; she was going to do the lying. She was not going to be manipulated; she was going to become a skillful manipulator. She was not going to be hurt by anyone; she would now do the hurting. These conscious choices were now the driving force behind Lucy's unconscious behavior. She identified with and became like her early life oppressors.

By carefully listening and paying attention to Lucy, Joe came to recognize that her words and actions continually displayed varying levels of anger, blame, and hatred. When she wasn't being overtly hateful, her passive aggressive behavior and words were covertly hostile. Joe began to see that Lucy rarely missed an opportunity to act upon her hatred of him.

Finally, by his improved understanding of the complex dynamic that was taking place in regard to his relationship with Lucy, and how it was related to his past trauma and present night terrors, Joe finally began to figure out how to overcome and cope with his marital challenges. This necessary first step, a comprehension of healthy and unhealthy parental and spousal relationships, later led to some workable solutions to his night terror problem.

While many books on parental relationships and child abuse helped Joe to sort out his distorted perceptions about his parents, most spousal relationship books were not very helpful in increasing Joe's understanding of Lucy. None of them really dealt with persons like her. Lucy's level of dysfunction far exceeded the scope of these works. However, the books that dealt with adults without conscience, psychopaths, "people of the lie," and trust bandits described Lucy on almost every page.

At the beginning of this section, I asked if the similarity between Joe's wife and his parents was a coincidence. It wasn't. Dr. Peck sometimes refers to these types of psychopaths as "evil." That's a very subjective term that has only recently become more widely used and conceptualized since the events of 9/11. But Peck answered my initial question when stating: "It is extraordinary how well the evil fit the mold. Once you've seen one evil person, you've essentially seen them all." (2, p.264)

Joe's case study is exceptionally relevant to an understanding of the diagnosis and treatment of Type B Night Terrors. Therefore, it will be discussed further in the next chapter. The last stages of his case history will be presented in chapter 13.

Chapter 11

The Psychopath Connection

The *Diagnostic Statistical Manual (DSM IV)* states the following:

"The essential feature of Antisocial Personality Disorder is a pervasive pattern of disregard for, and violation of, the rights of others that begins in childhood or early adolescence and continues into adulthood. This pattern has also been referred to as *psychopathy* . . . Deceit and manipulation are [the] central features."

"[Psychopaths] show little remorse for the consequences of their acts. They may be indifferent, [or] blame the victims, or provide a superficial rationalization for having hurt, mistreated, or stolen from someone (e.g., 'losers deserve to lose' or 'he had it coming anyway')."

"Appears to be associated with low socioeconomic status, [and] may be underdiagnosed in females, particularly because of the emphasis on aggressive items in the definition of [this] disorder."

"Lack of empathy, inflated self-appraisal, and superficial charm are features that have been commonly included in traditional conceptions of psychopathy . . . These individuals may also be irresponsible and exploitative in their sexual relationships. They may have a history of many sexual partners and may never have sustained a monogamous relationship." (3, pp.465, 466, 467)

Magid and McKelvy agreed with the above: "The mark of a

psychopath is habitual lying. It seems easier for them to lie than to tell the truth, and lying is done usually to try to persuade a person or to try to make the psychopath feel better at the moment." (38, p.17)

The first thing anyone should look at when evaluating a Type B Night Terror sufferer is his or her home situation. Lucy could not possibly stay married to anyone except Joe. Lucy is a psychopath. Joe was exposed to and tolerated psychopaths for his entire life prior to therapy. He spent his entire childhood appeasing and getting along with them. Because of his background, he was emotionally numb. His capacity to feel pain was drastically impaired; *that's the only thing that allowed him to survive his childhood.* The numbness, resistance to pain, and emotional blindness were a plus during childhood. The same traits become fatal when choosing a mate.

None of the doctors or therapists who encountered Joe and Lucy during their marriage recognized that Lucy was a psychopath. This is predominately because her mask of sanity and her act were flawless. The psychopath's ability to appear totally normal is a big part of the problem with the entire subject of Type B Night Terrors and also the reason that many practitioners still cling to their theories about genetic predisposition when encountering the victims of such consummate pretenders.

Many times, psychopaths are on both ends of this equation and the Type B Night Terror sufferer is in the middle. Joe's parents were both psychopaths. The woman he eventually married was a psychopath. Every time he went for help with his night terrors (both in childhood and adulthood) his history, along with his present circumstances, was being related to the doctor by a dedicated psychopath. Is it any wonder that the doctors who were trying to treat Joe found themselves completely in the dark? Magid and McKelvy stated that "[the psychopath] can lie with more confidence than you can tell the truth. Conning, slandering, and verbally manipulating others is what [they] do best." (38, p.337)

In childhood, Joe's Type B Night Terror attacks were so frequent and severe that others, besides his parents, were aware of the problem. This forced his parents to *pretend* to seek professional help. But seeking help was a ruse. They had no intention of telling any professional a single word of truth about the abuse they perpetrated on Joe.

Consider any doctor's position. Before him is a night terror sufferer (Joe). The doctor is aware of the school of thought that says night terrors are genetic. Joe's history is being told to the doctor by his parents. The doctor has no idea that he's dealing with dedicated psychopaths. They both come across as being the salt of the earth. They describe their home life as ideal, their marriage as blissful, and their commitment, love, and devotion to their son as exemplary. Putting on a show and manipulating people is what these two people do best. Any questions the doctor asks about possible negativity in the home are answered untruthfully by the parents. The portrait of a loving, tranquil home is being verbally painted by a pair of Rembrandts. The people in front of the doctor are consummate deceivers. Magid and McKelvy also stated, "Most therapists dread having to deal with the psychopath. Using their innate charm, psychopaths can con well-intentioned professionals." (38, p.x)

Joe's family doctor didn't have a chance of seeing through these people. First of all, he really had no reason to believe that they were lying. Since the doctor already believed that all night terrors are genetic, the peaceful home illusion and wonderful parents were consistent with that accepted scenario.

The doctor's assessment would certainly have been different if the parents had walked into his office and admitted, "From birth, we have maliciously beaten and tortured Joe at every opportunity." Unfortunately, and obviously, the abusive parents would never have confessed to anything like that. If they had, then doctors would have had good reason to look at the Chowchilla study, the Holocaust survivors, tortured POWs, and all other trauma-related night terrors, and be able to make the obvious connections.

Down the road, a similar scenario took place. Joe married

Lucy. Then the doctor began hearing about Joe's night terrors through her. Lucy was a master at extracting pity. All the doctor heard was, "Joe leaps up screaming, wakes me up, and has hurt me a couple of times. Oh doctor, I'm so scared and I don't know what to do. I love Joe so much." She then assured the doctor that the home is peaceful and loving, and the doctor concluded that Joe's night terrors were genetic.

Again, the doctor's assessment would certainly have been different if Lucy had walked in and told the truth. Suppose she had said, "I've been hating, using, and lying to Joe since the day we met." Unfortunately, Lucy would never have confessed to anything like that. If she had, the doctor would immediately have seen the connection between Joe's home life and the increase in his Type B Night Terror symptoms.

Joe's doctors remained in the dark. First his parents and years later Lucy had a vested interest in not telling the truth. The truth never came to the surface. The doctors were instead fed a slew of blatant lies. How then could medical professionals possibly have made any sense out of Joe's Type B Night Terrors?

Further complicating an accurate evaluation and assessment of the home is the fact that the great majority of young night terror sufferers are suffering from the Type A variety. Therefore, the great majority of parents are telling the truth about the home being peaceful and loving. The parents who are telling the truth seem exactly like the parents who are lying. In fact, the abusive psychopath may actually appear to be the most exemplary parent of them all. So suspecting abuse in all cases is certainly not the answer. The greatest travesty and injustice would be if the pendulum swung in the other direction, that is, if every doctor began thinking of abuse first in all childhood night terror cases.

Then what is the answer? Part of it is for doctors to keep these ideas in mind and pay careful attention. If a person still has night terrors once he or she reaches adulthood, then he most likely has the Type B variety and the professional needs to pay extremely careful attention to the people who are presenting the sufferer's story. If it's the parents, the doctor needs to ask how far back the night terrors go. If it turns out that the problem goes back to childhood, then he or she needs to ask why help wasn't sought back then. The sufferer's history has to be followed all the way back to birth if there is to be any hope of uncovering the truth.

A significant article in which the parents related inaccurate facts about their son, a nine-year-old night terror sufferer, shows how two doctors saw through the lies by carefully and objectively scrutinizing the situation over time. In that article, Dr. Garland and Dr. Smith wrote: "While a family history of psychiatric disorder was initially denied, the mother subsequently reported social anxiety and alcohol abuse in the child's maternal grandfather. . . . Precipitants for the onset of the night terrors and panic attacks were initially denied. It became clear over time, however, that serious covert marital problems were occurring, including extramarital affairs on the part of the child's father and an in-home separation of the parents, not discussed with the children, in which the father moved to a separate bedroom." (25, p.554)

First, the mother had blatantly lied about any family history of psychiatric disorders. But, because Dr. Garland and Dr. Smith pressed the issue, eventually some truth had come out. The mother had subsequently reported that there was some family history of psychiatric disorder. Next, both she and the father had lied about the situation within their home. They had initially denied anything aberrant going on in their household that could possibly be putting their child on edge or making him apprehensive before bedtime. Again, because the doctors pressed the issue, over time their attention to detail paid off. It turned out that there was a huge amount of dysfunction in the home that everyone was covering up.

If the doctors had not been observant, persistent, and willing to keep their focus on the situation "over time," they would not have seen through the initial lies of the parents. If they had believed the parents' story and then concluded that there was no prior or present family dysfunction, assuming the child's night terrors to be genetic, they would have been on the wrong track. Prior and present family dysfunction was definitely part of this child's problem.

Second, had the parents been more accomplished and convincing liars, the truth about their home might not have surfaced. If they had been polished psychopaths, capable of lying more convincingly than most people can tell the truth, even these two careful, conscientious doctors might not have been able to see through the deception.

These situations and evaluations are difficult. But for the professional practitioner, paying very careful attention to detail, and then carefully assessing the situation over time are definitely two important parts of the answer. Also, learning a little something about psychopaths in general will help.

Time is the only thing that can unmask a polished psychopath. This was demonstrated in Joe's case. No one, professional or otherwise, recognized that his parents and wife were psychopaths of the most dangerous kind. Joe's parents and Lucy combined the psychopathic characteristics of violence with self-delusion and the pretense of innocence. Recognizing the parent or spouse who is a psychopath has always been difficult. However, these types of people should become easier to detect and unmask once the practitioners fully understand the typical relationship between the Type B Night Terror sufferer and the psychopath. Also, when professionals come to accept that such night terrors are caused by extreme trauma they will know better what to look for, both in terms of the sufferer's repressed emotions and the psychopath connection. They will then surely pursue their investigation with greater thoroughness than did Joe's doctors.

Joe's night terrors would have been resolved long ago if only the professionals he saw had understood that Type B Night Terror sufferers are often chosen by dysfunctional psychopaths. With this realization it should take only a reasonable measure of caution and patient observation to determine if a spouse is like Lucy. Magid and McKelvy stated, "Despite the initial charm of these individuals, it is hard to confuse the *long-term* pattern of be-havior of a psychopath with anything else." (38, p.13) In other words, in most cases, time will eventually betray even the smoothest psychopath if a doctor is steadfast, determined, and knows what to look for.

In the past, Joe's doctors were deceived by his parents, and later on by his wife. Someone besides Joe was always in the room telling the story. But, as an adult, he could have answered questions and spoken for himself. Since it would not be terribly un-common for the Type B Night Terror sufferer to be involved in an abusive relationship, Joe should have been interviewed alone. He might not have been able to answer honestly if Lucy was sitting in the same room. She could have been interviewed separately. A mature night terror sufferer should always be interviewed in pri-vate.

It might also have been revealing to first interview Joe alone and then interview him together with Lucy. Rather than pay at-tention to her words during the second interview, the doctor should have then paid attention to see if Joe's demeanor or an-swers changed in any way. Suppose he noticed that Joe went from being calm when talking alone to being tense when talking with Lucy in the room, or, maybe, from being verbally open to care-fully watching his words, or, possibly, from hinting that things were wrong to enthusiastically declaring his home life to be won-derful. In those cases the doctor might have begun to suspect something strange about Lucy and their marriage. Unfortunately, most truths about Type B Night Terror sufferers must be ascer-tained through the back door. It must be assumed that there will be mostly distortion when going in through the front door.

Another important point is for the doctor to pay careful atten-tion to the words of the night terror sufferer and be ready to ask for more detail. These sufferers downplay everything. They are also prone to agree with whatever their parents and/or spouse says. They've gotten along with these people by being yes-men or yes-women. The doctor should make a point of thoughtfully extracting more information on anything even remotely suspect. Of course, he or she is highly unlikely to get the sufferer to reveal any details while the parents and/or spouse are present.

Dr. Peck kept pressing for details about one of his own anxiety disorder patients. George had initially reported that his sex life was fine and nothing was terribly wrong with his wife, outside of a little moodiness. The doctor later discovered that the extent of George and Gloria's "fine sex life" was one drunken quickie about every month and a half, and that her moodiness lasted for weeks at a time. He described Gloria as "significantly depressed [and] filled with hatred for George." (2, p. 23)

George had also initially downplayed his highly dysfunctional and violent childhood home. Dr. Peck took nothing at face value. He did not accept the easily acquired information and did not opt for the quick and easy solution of simply prescribing anxiety drugs.

A further important point is to pay attention to the verbal content of the night terror attack. If the sufferer screams words about his or her spouse during a night terror attack, that may be a red flag. It could simply be because the spouse is the only one in the bedroom when they are asleep. But it might be an extremely repressed sufferer acting out what he really feels about his spouse during the day. As is true in many Type B Night Terror cases, it could be the individual's subconscious talking. In that case, the sleeping sufferer's finger could be pointing directly at his present problem.

Finally, the doctor should make sure that the "identified patient" is really the person he or she should be studying as the cause of the patient's Type B Night Terrors. Since Joe had the night terrors, he was always the identified patient, even though others in his life were, psychologically, sicker than he was. Because of his night terrors it was mistakenly assumed that he was the least psychologically healthy person involved.

What happened to Joe in seeking treatment is probably similar to the experiences of other Type B Night Terror sufferers. In childhood, no help was offered. The treating professional believed the fictitious story presented by Joe's parents, assumed that

Joe suffered from pure childhood Type A Night Terrors, and told them that he would probably outgrow the condition. The parents were completely satisfied with that answer because it meant that there would be no investigation into the malicious abuse that they were perpetrating on Joe.

What happened later in life was even worse. Lucy insisted that Joe get professional help. She not only presented a completely inaccurate story to the doctor, but worse yet, Lucy essentially demanded that the professional address *her* sleeping problem, not Joe's. She wanted to be able to sleep at night without being awakened, but she wanted nothing about their miserable marriage known or addressed. Not surprisingly, getting some undisturbed sleep for Lucy became the focal point of the intervention.

In the throes of a night terror attack, while in stage four sleep, Joe's subconscious had been screaming out about his past and present emotional pain. But regrettably, after only a fifteen-minute consultation in which Lucy did all the talking, the doctor prescribed a relatively high dosage of a benzodiazepine drug. As will be discussed in the chapter on solutions, these drugs suppress deep, slow wave stage four sleep. Since night terrors occur in this stage of sleep, the curtailing of it works to reduce the symptoms.

Although Joe's night terror symptoms predictably did diminish, none of his deep-seated underlying problems were being addressed or solved. In addition, the taking of the drug created a new problem. By suppressing stage four sleep, benzodiazepine drugs essentially nullify that vital and necessary requirement for daily functioning. After spending a lifetime with Type B Night Terrors, sufferers are usually able to learn how to function reasonably well because the night terrors merely interrupt a portion of their stage four sleep. However, they can no longer function effectively in daily life when drugs virtually eliminate that vital stage of sleep.

By diminishing Joe's stage four sleep, the benzodiazepine drugs caused disruptions in the formerly functional areas of his life. Even with night terrors, Joe had been a good father, a conscientious driver, a competent worker, a proficient family financial manager, and a mostly functional individual. Over a lifetime, he had learned to compartmentalize his dysfunction. Only his emotional life was awry. Now, since he was getting almost no stage four sleep, not only were his past and present emotional problems not being addressed, the functional areas of his life were also falling apart. His patience and involvement with his children suffered, he drove around the freeways in a sleep-deprived daze, and his work performance and absenteeism became job-threatening concerns. The sudden inability to perform successfully in these formerly highly functional areas was adding a huge amount of pressure to Joe's already highly stressed life. Additionally, Joe's night terrors during stage four sleep had been his only previous outlet for his repressed emotions, which now exploded into his entire waking life.

Yes, Joe's night terror symptoms were lessened by the high dosages of the drug. He wasn't waking Lucy up as much. Her sleeping life was becoming better while Joe's waking, sleep-deprived life was becoming immeasurably worse. As a result, Lucy thanked the doctor for "solving" Joe's night terror problem and canceled their scheduled follow-up appointments. She was quite satisfied with the medical intervention.

However, Joe wasn't at all satisfied. He was able to realize how much worse his life had become because of the drugs. Of course! The initial fifteen-minute professional consultation yielded only a Band-Aid solution to what was a deep and complicated thirty-year problem. As I will detail in the chapter on solutions, decades old night terror problems require more than a superficial quick fix.

On his own, Joe decided to discontinue the medication. He concluded that he was better off with night terrors than with no sleep. Lucy was furious with Joe's "selfish and inconsiderate" decision. She demanded that Joe sleep in another room so that he didn't wake her up. She had considered drugs the perfect answer.

But this type of hasty intervention is harmful, not helpful. Joe's true problems needed to be the focus of careful, knowledgeable investigation. Then appropriate treatment should have been initiated. The lies of parents and/or spouses must not continue to dictate the course of action professionals take and must not continue to influence their concept of successful intervention. Lucy was able to prevail because night terror sufferers characteristically lack the assertiveness to confront and possibly anger someone in the process of finding effective solutions to their problems.

In attempting to detect and understand psychopaths, I strongly recommend the book *High-Risk: Children Without a Conscience*, by Magid and McKelvy. I believe that the first hundred pages should be required reading for every Type B Night Terror sufferer and every professional who deals with this subject. There are common traits that appear almost universally among these people. If you understand one psychopath, you probably will be better able to recognize, understand, and deal with others like him/her. In the above mentioned book Magid and McKelvy wrote:

"In some cases, the [unattached] child may learn that he cannot trust others and others will not care for him. Consequently, he fails to learn to care for others and to develop a conscience. (38, p.61).

"These people, more commonly known as psychopaths, express no remorse when caught in wrongdoings. They are aggressive, reckless and cruel to others. They leave in their wake a huge amount of human suffering. The pain psychopaths wreak on other human beings can be physical, or it can be *mental anguish often felt by those who try to form relationships with psychopaths.*" (38, p.3)

"The marriages of these people often involve physical and verbal fighting . . . Sexual promiscuity is common . . . [They are] socially isolated without any true friends." (38, pp.6, 7)

"Trust, love, loyalty, and teamwork are incompatible with their way of life. They scorn and exploit most people who are kind, trusting, hard-working and honest." (38, p.9)

"Since no partner is valued, any one partner can be exchanged for any other; in the absence of love, there is no pain in loss." (38, p.63)

"Their mask of sanity isn't real, but they often are so good at playing the part that at first their victims don't realize they are being manipulated." (38, p.85)

"Mr. and Mrs. Wrong cheat on their mates . . . lie whenever it suits them and sometimes even resort to violence. *Often marriages occur before the truth surfaces.*" (38, p.307)

In *People of The Lie*, Dr. M. Scott Peck also commented on the same kinds of people as follows:

"The words 'image,' 'appearance,' and 'outwardly' are crucial to understanding the morality of evil. While they seem to lack any motivation to be good, they intensely desire to appear good . . . not so much to deceive others *as to deceive themselves*. They cannot or will not tolerate the pain of self-reproach." (2, p.75) Peck went on to explain that the surreptitiously evil have at least a minimum concept of right and wrong or a "rudimentary form of conscience," otherwise they would not find it necessary to lie. People lie to cover up what they know or suspect to be wrong. (2, p.75)

"Because they are such experts at disguise, it's seldom possible to pinpoint the maliciousness of the evil." (2, p.76)

Dr. Chu's book *Rebuilding Shattered Lives,* is not about psychopaths, trust bandits, or people of the lie. It's about troubled people who seek professional help, something psychopaths rarely do. Nevertheless, one section of his book deals with adults who have backgrounds very similar to Lucy's. These victims of childhood sexual abuse become "chronically disempowered" adults. What makes these people stand out, even among the most difficult of Chu's patients, is not only their habit of abusing and exploiting others, but their strong tendency to be "impervious to change." (34, p.181,182) He explained that in their view of the world, there is not even the possibility of internal or external change or growth. Other than "dysfunctional isolation" their only option is to continually reenact their abusive childhood by applying the same deceitful, angry script on everyone else, assuming that all will "grow to hate" them anyway. (34, p.183)

Chu explained: "Lacking the ability to engage with others in a collaborative way, chronically disempowered patients continue to rely on control and manipulation as ways of meeting their needs . . . Because it feels impossible to *trust enough* to do things with others, the only alternative is to *do things to others.*" (34, p.187)

It is important to realize that psychopaths are not at all uncommon. Dr. Peck wrote: "My own experience, however, is that evil human beings are *quite common and usually appear quite ordinary to the superficial observer.* Like it or not, the psychiatrist sees as much psychopathology at cocktail parties, conferences, and corporations as in his or her own office." (2, pp.47, 86) Magid and McKelvy concurred with Dr. Peck when writing, "Psychopaths possess a poisonous mix of traits. They are arrogant, shameless, immoral, impulsive, antisocial, superficial, charming, callous, irresponsible, irreverent, cunning, self-assured. They are found in jails and mental institutions, but they can also be found in boardrooms or in politics or in any number of respected professions." (38, p.2)

The link between exposure to psychopaths and the development of Type B Night Terrors is also not unprecedented. All of the Auschwitz survivors developed some level of Type B Night Terrors. The Nazis who ran the camps as well as the guards who carried out this extreme brutality had some degree of psychopathology. What's even more amazing is how common psychopathology may really be. The Nazis had no trouble finding people who could be talked into accepting the dehumanization, brutalization, and extermination of fellow humans. Almost an entire nation (as well as many occupied nations) went along with it. The sheer number of those who enthusiastically and wholeheartedly carried out their gruesome duties is absolutely astounding. Dedicated psychopaths were everywhere!

Are they any less common today? One has only to look at the aftermath of any modern ethnic conflict to realize that there are many psychopaths just waiting for an opportunity to come out of the woodwork and do some damage. Where are all these psychopaths hiding before racial cleansing, an ethnic war, or some other dehumanizing conflict brings them out? They are hiding in plain sight, in average looking homes and families.

Even in America, there is an alarming increase in evidence supporting Magid and McKelvy's suspicion that this nation, too, might be a "breeding ground for psychopaths." (38, p.1) While the vast majority of these deviants go undetected, a small percentage of them come to our attention through the media. However, before they become publicly known because of some heinous crime, these individuals have already exposed those who were attempting to establish interpersonal relationships with them to the common psychopathological traits detailed in this chapter. For example, *New York Times* reporters C. LeDuff and D. Murphy wrote the following about the beltway sniper, John Allen Muhammad: "Beneath the *veneer*, he was seen by some as a stalker and *fibber*, qualities that fit a *lifetime pattern of deceit* and tall tales—and *manipulative romances* with women." (66, p.15)

I hope, this chapter has helped you to recognize the psychopaths who may be in your own life, whether you are a night terror sufferer with a psychopath attempting to spin a web of lies around you, a medical or psychological professional dealing with night terror sufferers, or simply an interested reader. In any case, developing an awareness of the existence and traits of these types of people is an important step.

Chapter 12

Additional Proof of the Trauma Connection

Evidence from Munchausen by Proxy Videotapes and SIDS

One of the most glaring examples of how much damage can be done by deranged individuals wearing masks of sanity has only recently surfaced. The latest covert Munchausen by proxy syndrome videotape has graphically demonstrated how remarkably convincing of their total innocence some abusive parents can be. Videotape has captured disturbed mothers intentionally suffocating, poisoning, overmedicating, bruising, cutting, and breaking the bones of their own children. For decades, doctors had been ignoring what was clearly in front of their noses and had been sending these obviously abused and tortured children back home to be further tortured or even killed by their own mothers. The facts said one thing, and the mothers in question (tearful, cunning, consummately proficient manipulators and liars) said another.

The doctors had consistently chosen to believe the mothers over the facts. If it were not for video surveillance and the amazing recoveries the children in question experienced once they were removed from their mothers, the profession would probably still be the dupes of these perpetrators; after all, accepting the mother's account had always been the standard approach. But, with the evidence now available, the medical community is remorseful about having been deceived by these sick women, and about its complicity in this travesty. As Shannon Brownlee wrote:

"Once the ruse is uncovered, doctors and nurses are devastated to learn that they unwittingly have served as child abusers." (44, p.59)

Well-intentioned professionals had been blindly playing a role in the abuse and death of these tortured children because they were mistaking the mothers' proficient storytelling for truth and subsequently ruling out other possibilities. The most stubborn and resistant barrier to truth is the perception that one already has it.

Sharon Begley reinforced this same point when writing about the devastating effects of an influential article on sudden infant death syndrome (SIDS) that prevented pediatricians and researchers from considering abuse in such cases for over twenty-five years. She wrote: "Alfred Steinschneider argued that SIDS runs in families and is caused by prolonged sleep apnea. The paper became an instant classic." A quarter century later, the journal that had published this article expressed remorse: "We should never have published this article. Some physicians still believe SIDS runs in families. It doesn't— murder does." (45, p.72)

In addition, Kathryn Godfrey wrote that "attacks are usually carried out on children *under the age of 20 months*." (46, p.24) And Shannon Brownlee reported: "Adults victimized by a parent with MBP [later] suffered from *post traumatic stress disorder* (PTSD) symptoms similar to those of other victims of traumatic events." (44, p.59)

Although the proof of what was happening to these children had been there for decades, it took videotaped evidence to firmly make the point that "a mother" is not necessarily a universal constant or synonym for love and concern. Timely truth and timely recognition are what benefits the most vulnerable: the infants who cannot speak out or defend themselves.

Munchausen by proxy syndrome videotapes also revealed that intentional suffocation is the number one act perpetrated upon infants by Munchausen syndrome mothers. David Southall wrote: "CVS revealed abuse in 33 of 39 suspected cases, with documentation of intentional suffocation observed in 30 patients.

Poisonings, a deliberate fracture, and other emotional and physical abuse were also identified under surveillance." (47, p.96) Donald, Jureidini, and DeAngelis reported something similar when writing: "In the late 1970s, case reports appeared of infants with apnea, apparently induced by their mothers' suffocation of them. Perhaps the abusive parent is in some way gratified and excited by almost killing the baby and witnessing its subsequent return to life." (48, p.757) A. Souid and associates wrote: "Children in such cases have been infected, bled, poisoned, suffocated, starved and otherwise abused by a parent who thrives on the attention that caring for the child brings them." (49, p.497)

Evidence from Typical Type B Night Terror Cases

In the area of Type B Night Terrors, there is still a lack of perception and recognition of the true causes of the problem, as was the case prior to the official recognition of the causes of Munchausen by proxy. But, the evidence against erroneous points of view keeps on mounting.

As mentioned earlier, most of the night terror literature talks about almost all Type B Night Terror victims experiencing similar "dreams" during terror episodes. They are in a panic because they are being *suffocated, choked, dying, or escaping something.* For years I have been asking people in the sleep field to explain why they think it is that night terror victims are all having similar "dreams." If night terrors are a genetically caused condition, then it makes absolutely no sense that almost all the sufferers are having the same kinds of dreams during an attack, and that being suffocated is the number one recollection in an astounding number of cases.

Throughout the decades night terror literature overflows with the same observations. Susan Knapp wrote that the mental content accompanying most night terrors is "a single frightening feeling or sensation such as falling, *choking,* being crushed, etc." (5, p.181) Dr. Kales wrote: "The fright displayed during a night ter- ror event gives the impression that the person is trapped and is desperately fighting back while *being attacked.*" (13, p.1416) Dr. Williams noted that: "Classic features of the night terrors include pre-arousal impressions of fear, *choking* and impending doom." (50, p.135)

The Munchausen by proxy videotapes, evidence gleaned from SIDS, the *JAMA* report's proof of chemical changes in the brain as a result of abuse—together with our advanced understandings of traumatic dreams and nightmares—now make a concrete con- nection between the choking, suffocating dreams of many Type B Night Terror sufferers and past infant trauma. The sequence of events and repercussions are at last painfully clear. Trauma re- sulting from severe abuse is clearly the cause of the later Type B Night Terror attacks that often develop in victims.

In general, the traumatic dream is the domain of unresolved anxiety, emotional concerns, and stress. Such stress is so intense that the defensive waking repression will not even allow the indi- vidual an awareness of it, much less allow the person to attempt to resolve it. This gets replayed in the subconscious, a safe place, in an attempt to master and make connections about it, because it is a kind of stress that is too intense to be accessible when the in- dividual is awake.

The traumatic recurring dream that typically happens during Type B Night Terrors is partially an expression of the outraged and overwhelmed subconscious, partially a self-attempt at coping with an earlier anxiety or trauma, and partially an attempt to rewrite the sufferer's personal history. The victim is attempting to change an ending that happened decades ago by leaping out of his or her sleep at the point in the recurring night terror attack when the most painful and damaging trauma (such as suffoca- tion) is about to take place. The actual content of the night terror consists of the sufferer envisioning him- or herself fighting back before the trauma occurs in the so-called dream. While asleep, the victim is fleeing, fighting, wrestling, resisting the person who had attempted to abuse him or her decades before when he or she lacked the physical ability and/or awareness to resist. But sadly, try as the victim might, he or she can make very little headway. The past cannot be changed. That is why the Type B Night Terror "dream" continues to be replayed for decades in the deepest stages of sleep.

Until recently, few connections, explanations, or outside validation could be offered to the sufferer. A psyche, entrapped in the perceptual world of one who is in a helpless situation (such as that of an infant), was left to wrestle with this enormous emotional monster, alone! Yet, forty years ago, long before the above was documented, Dr. Leo Eitinger and others noted that there would be no change in the condition until the trauma was validated and dealt with and conscious connections were made by the sufferer. Susan Knapp also knew that the content of the traumatic night terror was an attempt to master a stress and rewrite the ending. She noted that once therapists dealt with the cause and effect relationship between the Chowchilla kidnapping and the night terrors of the school-age victims, many symptoms abated.

Even when dealing with lower level stresses, the resolution process is directly tied to making connections. Dr. Hartmann studied three women who were having recurring nightmares after undergoing abortions: "The dreams stopped entirely after the women made the connection with the abortion and dealt with it in some way. One of these women said that the simple realization that the dreams were related to guilt about the abortion was enough to stop the dreams." (27, p.72)

As many researchers understood and wrote about for decades, Type B Night Terror sufferers needed to have their psychologists and psychiatrists validate their trauma. They needed help in deciphering the meaning of the content and events of the recurring night terrors. Then they required professional help to effectively cope, address the anxiety, and make waking connections. Finally, they needed help in recognizing and addressing related circumstances, secondary complications, and far-reaching negative lifelong offshoots.

Unfortunately, Type B Night Terror sufferers have been receiving the exact opposite of what they have needed for healing. Attributing the condition to genetics negated and dismissed the trauma. Trying to convince the patient that the content of the night terror attack was meaningless added to the individual's repression, anxiety, and inability to make waking sense out of any part of his or her past, present, and future. Trauma-related offshoots were not even considered. Therefore, no meaningful coping, anxiety allaying, or connection-making assistance was available. Thus, night terrors became a life sentence.

Workable solutions are available. But they all begin with an accurate understanding and recognition of the initial trauma, the manifestations that develop as a result, and the numerous spiraling and escalating offshoots.

In summary, the proof of the trauma connection to Type B Night Terrors is now clear. The present and prior chapters have covered the subject in detail and provide the necessary background for the conscientious reader to be able to understand and effectively apply the solutions discussed in the next chapter.

Chapter 13

Solutions for Type B Night Terrors

[My suggestions for dealing with Type A Night Terrors were contained in chapter 5, which explained ways to deal with them. In order to avoid any confusion, I did not put those answers in this section. This chapter is exclusively about solutions to Type B Night Terrors. Information from earlier in the book will now be coordinated with solutions to the many problems and offshoots arising from Type B Night Terrors.]

What Is a Real Cure?

For some time there have been both harmful and relatively harmless drugs available for dealing with only the actual Type B Night Terror symptoms. Neither category of drug has addressed the true core of the problem. Instead, the drugs were a quick, short-sighted attempt to limit the frequency and severity of the disruptive night terror attack itself. In 1994, Lillywhite, Wilson, and Nutt published an article in the *British Journal of Psychiatry* entitled "Successful Treatment of Night Terrors and Somnambulism with paroxetine (Paxil)." paroxetine does not constitute a cure for the ongoing psychological problems at the root of Type B Night Terrors, but it often masks the symptoms without the drastic side effects of the more widely used benzodiazepine drugs. In their article, Lillywhite and associates questioned the use of the benzodiazepine drugs. Since these "suppress slow wave sleep" and therefore have a devastating effect on the sufferer's waking life, researchers found that "anti-panic" drugs such as paroxetine, routinely used to treat anxiety disorders, were more effective for night terrors and had fewer side effects than the benzodiazepines. (51, p.553)

As stated in an earlier chapter, the benzodiazepines essentially disrupt and limit stage four sleep, the deep sleep in which night terrors occur. Unfortunately, that stage of sleep is necessary for normal waking functioning. This approach is like attempting to cure loud snoring by waking up the snoring person every time he begins to fall asleep. Granted, the snoring would be virtually eliminated, but that solution would prevent the sufferer from getting any restful sleep. Similarly, benzodiazepines reduce the incidence of night terror attacks only because they reduce the amount of stage four sleep that the sufferer experiences. So while these drugs are intermittently or temporarily successful in reducing night terror activity, the patient becomes severely sleep deprived. Thus, the victim is left in a waking stupor due to the lack of stage four sleep. He or she can also become vulnerable to all the physical ailments that stem from lack of sleep.

Lillywhite and associates found that paroxetine was effective in reducing the incidence of night terror attacks without the patient experiencing stupor. It had long been known that anxiety-reducing drugs benefited Type B Night Terror sufferers. But, why these drugs were effective in treating what was widely believed to be a genetic, non-anxiety related disorder was unclear. Carlson and White put the obvious pieces together back in 1982 when writing: "This raises the possibility that night terrors are, in fact, an anxiety disorder, it is interesting to note that the medications frequently used to treat persons with acute anxiety have also been found to be effective in the treatment of night terrors." (20, p.466)

We now know exactly why these drugs were effective. The

JAMA report stated: "In rats many of the neurobiological conse-quences of [stress], including CRF hypersecretion, are *reversed* by treatment with antidepressants, including *paroxetine* (Paxil)." (4, p.596). The positive benefit of paroxetine in the treatment of night terrors is no longer unexplained, speculative, or mystifying. Extreme abuse early in life results in brain chemistry changes that precipi-tate the onset of anxiety disorders such as night terrors. And drugs like paroxetine, which allay acute anxiety, do so by reversing the CRF hypersecretion responsible for the individual's anxiety disor-der symptoms.

Therefore, paroxetine definitely fits into some phase of the treatment of Type B Night Terrors—but which phase? In the past, all drugs, even paroxetine, have served to mask the night terror symptoms and have precluded and prevented anyone from ad-dressing or dealing with the true issues of the sufferer. As men-tioned earlier, Wilise Webb accurately wrote: "No amount of [drugs] will cure the troubled mind. Unless time, circumstances, or our own efforts have removed the pressures which require the use of the drug, those pressures will continue; they have been only tem-porarily masked." (7, pp.126, 127) Dr. Chu concurred with Webb when writing: "Medications should not be the primary therapeu-tic interventions." (34, p.168) He added, "benzodiazepines are usually of limited effectiveness over time." (34, p.168)

Most professionals agree that their job entails more than sim-ply making a hasty diagnosis and then administering drugs. Why, then, has this been the standard course of action if any treatment at all was offered to Type B Night Terror sufferers? Because of a lack of awareness. Had psychiatric and psychological profession-als been aware that they were dealing with extreme, unresolved earlier trauma, lifelong health and personality difficulties, and current interpersonal or marital problems, most conscientious practitioners would have attempted to address these issues. Instead, either nothing was done or drugs comprised the totality of therapeutic intervention.

If, as is likely, the night terror victim was in an extremely dys-functional marriage, the drugs, when effective, allowed the individual to sleep through the issues that the subconscious had been screaming about at night. Additionally, they prevented any therapeutic benefit from coming out of the connections that the sufferer's subconscious was trying to make about the almost certain traumatic earlier experiences, and also precluded any professional from dealing with both of these issues while the sufferer was awake.

Earlier in the book, Dr. Hartmann explained the essential role that dreams play in mastering stresses (27, p.125). Unless the issues are addressed, the drugs not only mask the symptoms, they bind and gag the subconscious, the only part of the repressed night terror sufferer capable of speaking out on his or her own behalf. The drugs also do away with the only part of the individual that is aware of, and attempting to deal with or master extreme unresolved stresses. Only in the deepest stages of sleep, during the night terror attack, is the sufferer facing the truth about his or her past and present painful emotional realities. Therefore, dealing with the symptoms merely by giving the sufferer drugs does not resolve anything; rather, it paints over these deep and complicated problems.

On top of this, when drugs are the only solution, the physical health problems associated with Type B Night Terrors are not being addressed either. On the contrary, the additional stress and turmoil that the drugs add to the night terror sufferer's life may lead to further deterioration in the patient's health. Thus, this approach is not truly therapeutic. As mentioned earlier, the only real beneficiary might be a dysfunctional, abusive spouse who can now sleep through the night.

Suppose a woman who was severely abused in childhood were to develop lifelong Type B Night Terrors and then grow up and marry an abusive, violent man. Then suppose that this stress caused a latent explosion of night terror activity. Would this woman benefit if the totality of her treatment was the elimination of her night terror symptoms even with paroxetine? No! The drug would only address the most obvious and immediate manifestation: the night terror symptoms. Eliminating the symptoms would preclude anyone from dealing with her horrendous past and present problems. The words and actions during her night terror attacks would probably be directed at her husband. While asleep, she would be pointing to her present problem. If paroxetine were to be administered to this patient, then the nocturnal pointing would stop, but the abuse at the hands of her husband and the lifelong torment inside her psyche would continue.

Later Use of Paroxetine May Be Better

The manner in which the resolution of Joe's night terror problem was carried out represents the most effective sequence of therapeutic strategies yet devised for the treatment of Type B Night Terrors. It's a faster, more focused, and more direct approach to the decade long process and steps that I used to resolve my own night terrors. Even though Joe had been going to many therapists over the years, it was only with my step-by-step guidance that he was able to effectively cure himself of his lifelong night terrors. By the time he came to me, he was already convinced that his night terrors were trauma-related rather than of genetic origin. So, getting to the bottom of this traumatic cause became his top priority. He set about the task of finding out everything about his past and present, which eventually led to an understanding of how this information was related to his severe and virtually lifelong night terror attacks.

In the process that Joe went through, drugs were not tried until most of his night terror problem was already under control. During the early stages of treatment, he came to understand his underlying psychological problems as well as his past and present emotional turmoil. He was continually making connections and personal discoveries, sorting things out, unearthing long buried issues and growing in self-awareness.

It is this increased growth and awareness that eventually resulted in the diminution of Joe's night terror activity. A once chronic nightly problem dwindled down to only an occasional concern.

Almost constant violent night terror attacks were replaced by intermittent mild awakenings. Leaping out of sleep screaming and then running around the room eventually gave way to quietly sitting up in bed for a minute during his night terror episodes. By the mid-point of his treatment these mild episodes were occurring only several times a month rather than every night.

This discovery process was long, slow, detailed and arduous. But it was effective! Before Joe came to me, numerous therapists had helped him to explore his dysfunctional childhood. But, while these professionals excelled at dealing with his early life issues, they failed to effectively probe his present emotional life, and even more important, they made no connection between all these emotional issues and Joe's night terror problem. By combining the discoveries he had made in therapy with my own understandings about the early life causes, later offshoots, and the requirements for the resolution of night terrors, Joe began to grasp the entire complicated picture of his chronically flawed emotional life.

Finally, because Joe was able to make deep emotional connections about his past and present in his waking life, there was less need for him to wrestle with these issues at night. Because Joe came to recognize the dysfunction in his marriage, he was able to sidestep much of this stress while interacting with his wife by day, and he was able to sleep better by night.

Also, Joe stopped downplaying the impact of his childhood trauma on his later emotional decisions in life. His new perspective helped him to stop blaming himself entirely for his problems. This in itself was highly therapeutic. Dr. Chu found that even those patients who are fully aware of the extent to which they were abused in childhood often downplay the significant role it plays in their present lives, making no connections between its negative consequences and their present interpersonal or emotional problems. (34, pp.39, 203)

In addressing his abusive background in the cold light of truth and reality, Joe severed many superficial dysfunctional negative family ties. He found a *barometer* of self-reality through his children by asking himself: "If someone had beaten my child that severely for years, and was totally unrepentant, would I still associate with that person?" The answer of course was no. Joe began to entitle himself to dignity and respect from everyone with whom he chose to associate. He stopped making excuses for many of the angry, hateful individuals he had formerly tolerated and with whom he had wasted his time.

Interestingly, Joe did not sever his ties to Lucy. Joe's brother-in-law's non-night-terror-related anxiety attacks went away after he divorced Lucy's sister. So, it would have seemed that Joe's night terror problem might have subsided if he had divorced Lucy. But, unlike his brother-in-law, Joe had a deep, loving, involved relationship with his children which would have been disrupted if he left Lucy. And the closeness with his children added far more to his life and emotional well-being than his new reality-based interactions with Lucy, cautious though they were, were now taking away.

Whether because of bonding/attachment or other factors, whatever it was that allowed the abusive past of the Type B Night Terror sufferer to manifest itself in that manner—as opposed to severe clinical depression, psychopathology, or becoming an abuser him- or herself—the night terror sufferer seems to have the proclivity for becoming a competent, nonabusive parent. After spending an entire childhood watching perfect examples of what not to be as a parent, Joe had an outstanding grasp of what good parenting entailed. He gave more thought and effort to the subject than most people who are raised in normal homes. Dr. Chu told of people like Joe who became "exemplary parents." He wrote that: "Some of our patients achieve a striking depth of character that has been forged through overcoming adversity." (34, pp.177, 208) Additionally, unlike most individuals who were severely abused in childhood, Joe was not only a competent, nonabusive, loving parent but a very trusting human being. This is also typical of Type B Night Terror sufferers.

In yet another irony, the same loving trust that made Joe such easy prey for Lucy also contributed to building a strong bond with his children, and that interpersonal bond was in itself highly therapeutic. In contrast, Lucy could not trust or build an honest bond with anyone, even her children. The building of trusted social supports provides the foundation for emotional healing. Dr. Chu reported that one of the most devastating consequences of severe childhood abuse, especially sexual abuse, is that its victims later are unable to take the emotional risks necessary to achieve the kind of trust that is usually associated with normal relationships. (34, pp. 49, 50)

The trusting, open relationship that Joe had with his children also served to ground Joe in reality. Grounding was an effective therapeutic technique for him. This is where the sufferer is led to envision someone he loves having to experience the kind of abuse that he or she has endured. As is common with abuse victims, Joe had a very disconnected and nonchalant way of looking at his abusive childhood. But one of his therapists would always ask him to envision one of his own children being brutalized in the same way that his parents had brutalized him. Just the thought of his children being abused was visibly painful and emotionally distressing for Joe. And yet, he could talk casually about the cruel things that happened to him without any emotion or reaction at all. Only through his children was he able to actually feel the ugly reality of his traumatic past and to integrate the feelings involved into his present emotional awareness. This led to the need for numerous adjustments in his life. As these were implemented, both Joe's internal and external stresses diminished and so did his incidence of night terror attacks.

Had I known about and told Joe about paroxetine when we first began talking, he might have taken this drug early on in order to limit or mask his chronic night terror symptoms. *In that case, we'd have interacted for a week instead of a year and none of these emotional resolutions and understandings would have surfaced.* Not only would the drug have prevented the emergence of emotional truth and reality in Joe's life, he would never have been able to gauge his progress.

Joe kept a log. He knew when he was on the right track in chasing down emotional concerns because of the drop-off in his night terror activity. When he was chasing the wrong tangents there was no change in his night terror activity. Also, he found that a phone call from one of his childhood abusers during the day would disturb his sleep that night. This affirmed the gut feeling he had always had about his parents. It helped him decide which relationships were detrimental to his long-term emotional health and would therefore have to be severed. Had he been taking paroxetine, he would have had no accurate way of measuring whether or not he was addressing the dominant past or present emotional concerns and no decision-making help regarding the people in his life.

When is the right time for the paroxetine? I'm sure every case will be different. But, after I pointed out the merits of the *JAMA* study, Joe went to Mexico and purchased the drug. He was not looking for a quick fix for his night terror problem; he'd already made headway toward a solution through taking the long, painful route. But, Joe was intrigued by the part of the *JAMA* study that talked about the drug "reversing the brain damage" from childhood. So he decided to try it in very low doses.

Joe cut the paroxetine pills into 10-milligram doses. This is far less than the minimum 20 milligrams per day that the *Physicians Desk Reference* recommends for treating all listed disorders, or the 40 milligrams per day that Lillywhite, Wilson and Nutt administered to the night terror patient in their study. (51, p.551) Experience has shown that most sufferers appear to benefit from 20 milligrams or more. However, patients need to consult a qualified professional for specific dosages. For Joe, deeper, more restful sleep resulted. Also, the very last of his night terror symptoms virtually disappeared. Those in which he would sit up in bed while asleep had still been occurring several times a month until then.

Recognizing, addressing, and dealing with his underlying past and present emotional concerns had been Joe's true path to achieving a dramatic reduction in his night terror symptoms. This should be the aim and approach in treating all Type B Night Terror sufferers. Only at the very end did Joe use paroxetine to smooth out the surface of an emotional hole that he had spent a lifetime filling up. Using the drugs later rather than earlier was definitely better for Joe.

It Takes Time and Effort

In this age of managed health care, fifteen-minute doctor visits, and a preference for the quick fix, the confirmed effectiveness of paroxetine in the treatment of night terror symptoms may prove to be more harmful than beneficial. The overall past and present emotional life of the sufferer, as well as the health and interpersonal concerns already addressed in this book, need to be dealt with before the administration even of such an effective drug as paroxetine. This is a long and involved process which can only be hindered by administering the drug.

For years, conscientious professionals have emphasized that many anxiety disorders can only be cured by the long process of addressing, coming to terms with, and making connections about deep past and present emotional issues. In regard to one of his own patients who was suffering from anxiety attacks, Dr. Peck wrote, *"Until you have dealt in much greater depth with your miserable marriage and your ghastly childhood, you're going to continue to be tortured by your symptoms."* (2, p.25) Exactly! All that is needed is for the same approach to be taken with Type B Night Terror sufferers. Now that it is finally recognized that Type B Night Terrors are an anxiety disorder, this therapeutic approach should be applicable in the great majority of cases.

The resolution of my own night terror problem, of Joe's, and of others I have observed, relied heavily on Dr. Peck's formula. Dr. Peck did not simply administer anxiety-reducing drugs. He resisted the quick fix, accepted the long-term challenge, and then set about doing some deep, intense, serious work. Addressing deep past and present emotional concerns should be the fundamental strategy in the war against Type B Night Terrors. This takes time, diligence, and patience.

Where to Start

How does one begin to address severe early trauma or any other severe past trauma, any related lifelong traumatic offshoots and health problems, numerous secondary complications, and any resultant interpersonal difficulties, as well as years of total inaction? The challenge is enormous! That's why I believe that all Type B Night Terror sufferers need a competent therapist to guide them through the steps that must be taken. Unfortunately, such sufferers cannot address issues to which they are blind, don't recognize, or have repressed and/or forgotten. They have too many areas of emotional blindness to attempt this journey alone. Also, it's very possible that the person(s) closest to the sufferer, such as the parents or spouse, may be a big part of the problem, and the sufferer will not recognize that without help.

Since right now there aren't too many therapists making a difference in the lives of night terror sufferers, how do you find a competent therapist? One of the main goals of this book is to begin the process of convincing professionals that the treatment of Type B Night Terrors needs to be approached in the same manner that they already utilize effectively in approaching many other anxiety disorders. Once they recognize Type B Night Terrors as an anxiety disorder, they already have the expertise to deal with this malady. The things the therapist must do in order to help the night terror sufferer are already part of his or her training, education, and practice. Most caring, conscientious therapists have the aptitude. All they need is a little direction in applying their expertise to the bizarre subject of night terrors. This book has enough answers and guidance for the professional to make a difference in the night terror sufferer's life.

If a patient is still suffering from night terrors well into adulthood, there should not be any more doubt that the condition almost certainly is trauma-related Type B Night Terrors. Therefore, the first step in treating this patient is the recognition that he or she is suffering from the same condition as the Auschwitz survivors, tortured POWs, survivors of marine disasters, various war veterans, the Chowchilla children, and many others. It should now be clear that the assumption of past extreme psychic trauma is a prerequisite for effective treatment.

In studying night terror sufferers, Leopold and Dillon noted: "As the long-term examination proceeded, the almost monotonous similarity of the psychological patterns was striking." (16, p.919) Informed generalities derived from these similarities have been found to be accurate in an astounding number of cases. Many other careful researchers have also noted this.

One can begin by assuming both extreme psychic trauma and/or abuse, in childhood or at some other time in the past, as well as present marital or extreme interpersonal dysfunction. Since the most recent studies prove that anxiety disorders on the level of night terrors result from abuse early in life, or at some past time in the life of the patient, the first assumption is not too bold. The assumption of interpersonal dysfunction is not very daring either. As discussed earlier, Eitinger found that severely traumatized people lose the capacity to make sensible marital and relationship decisions. This usually results in later interpersonal problems and stress.

Eitinger and others also noticed that the relatively few night terror sufferers who were lucky enough to acquire secure, peaceful interpersonal relationships suffered fewer night terror symptoms than those whose "hasty and injudicious" decisions landed them in highly dysfunctional marriages or other relationships. The very fact that a married sufferer might be seeking treatment at a particular time probably indicates that his or her symptoms are worse than they've been before. Otherwise, he or she would have sought treatment earlier. This explosion of latent symptoms is not only typical for sufferers but also indicative of some extreme unresolved present stress.

I saw this pattern in my own life. When I was involved in peaceful, loving adult relationships with sincere, emotionally healthy people, my night terror episodes were far less frequent and severe than when I was involved in volatile, unloving adult relationships with insincere, emotionally unhealthy people. During periods of peaceful adult relationships, I did not need to seek professional help. The night terror episodes were far less frequent and/or severe. It was only during the volatile adult relationships that I sought professional intervention because night terror explosions became a life disrupting nightly problem.

Another informed assumption would be that the night terror sufferer is completely blind to the angry type of abuser who can recognize and is actively targeting a spouse he or she can use and abuse. All the factors mentioned in chapter 9 make it highly likely that the night terror victim is involved in an extremely dysfunctional and stressful marriage or comparable relationship. *A functional, peaceful marriage or other relationship would be an aberration for a person who is suffering from frequent Type B Night Terrors.*

Without the assumptions set out above, one would not be able to effectively utilize Dr. Peck's realizations. Initially, in order to be able to deal with the psychological ramifications of one's "ghastly childhood" one must recognize that there was a ghastly childhood in the first place. Second, before dealing with a sufferer's "miserable marriage," one must be alert to the probability that extreme past psychic trauma may have left this individual emotionally numb and therefore quite likely to be in an extremely dysfunctional relationship.

It would also be helpful, but not necessary, to find out what the particular past trauma in question entailed. In many cases this will be impossible because many abuse victims forget whole segments of their childhood. However, therapists deal with past trauma and incomplete pictures all the time. A general understanding of the kind of severe and brutal childhood trauma necessary to produce Type B Night Terrors should be sufficient to begin addressing these issues. Sometimes the victim's recall about some of his or her night terror dreams may give hints about what the actual childhood abuse or other past trauma entailed, as in the numerous documented cases in which the dream involved being choked or choking. But, it can be assumed almost with a certainty that severe trauma had to have taken place in order to produce Type B Night Terrors, even if the exact details cannot be determined. So, there can be effective treatment even without establishing precisely what the particular past trauma entailed.

In asking about background, the therapist should be looking for possible past windows of opportunity where abuse might have taken place. It is surprising how many night terror patients were adopted, lived in foster homes, or were in situations where they were not with their natural parents sometime during their first years of life. Although such situations might be clues as to where the abuse might have taken place, the natural parents themselves can never be ruled out as the culprits, especially where the child was not really wanted or where the parents can be determined to have severe psychological problems themselves.

In observing and studying the patient per se, the therapist will usually discover that a few parts of the night terror sufferer's psyche are incredibly damaged, while most parts are remarkably intact. This is one of the fingerprints left behind by Type B Night Terrors. When the entire psyche has been horribly devastated, the patient is not a night terror sufferer; he or she is someone like Charles Manson or some other kind of psychopath. Careful questioning and painstaking attention to detail will reveal the gaping flaws in the night terror sufferer's background, psyche, and present emotional circumstances. By using the guidelines in this book, the careful professional should be able to sort out and solve many of the formidable puzzles and mysteries that envelop all night terror sufferers.

The Reliable Witness

Interviewing the night terror sufferer directly about his or her life may not be very helpful. However, if the verbal content that accompanies the night terrors is taken seriously, it may point to the problem. Numerous careful researchers have noted that the majority of Type B Night Terror sufferers experience dreams that usually have a consistent theme, one directly related to a past trauma or present stress. It should therefore not be surprising if the verbal content that accompanies the night terror attack turns out to contain some elements of truth. For example, if the sufferer is always verbally lashing out at the spouse during these attacks, this should be a clue that special attention needs to be paid to the spouse and the nature of the marital relationship.

The subconscious may be the only reliable witness. Everyone else could be either emotionally blind or lying. Night terror sufferers who were raised in an abusive home will probably not recognize their enemies while awake, but eventually the subconscious does react to the ongoing hatred and assault.

The revelations that may arise when the content of the night terrors is analyzed are another reason that paroxetine should not be administered at the beginning of therapy. If the subconscious is a truthful witness, and the sleeping night terror sufferer is pointing a finger at the past or present problem, then the drug will silence the only reliable witness upon which the treating professional can rely.

Six-Step Approach to Healing

Joe started out as a man with a chronic, out of control, lifelong Type B Night Terror problem that nothing, even medical intervention, had been able to alleviate prior to my sharing with him the understandings and solutions contained in this book. The implementation of much of the information I am now incorporating herein led to a steady decline in the frequency and severity of his night terror attacks. Over time, his once severe problem became only an intermittent concern, and then low-dose therapy with paroxetine virtually eliminated his scant remaining symptoms entirely. The key element in Joe's healing of his lifelong night terrors was the making of waking emotional connections about his past, his present, and himself. Throughout this book, Dr. Hartmann and other competent professionals have given valuable insights into this connection-making process and how it leads to healing.

The following is a quick overview of my observations, perceptions, and understandings about the steps that Joe took and the changes he instituted. These are essentially the same steps that I had initially taken in curing my own lifelong Type B Night Terrors, only they have been refined to be more effectively applied over a shorter period of time.

Step 1

The very first thing Joe did was to follow the guidelines that all sleep disorder sufferers, not just Type B Night Terror victims, should carefully adhere to. He eliminated all caffeine from his diet. People with sleep problems routinely ingest too much caffeine in an effort to compensate for their lack of sleep and remain productive during the day. The use of stimulants such as coffee, tea, and cola make solving any sleep problem nearly impossible. Although many troubled sleepers may be addicted to it, *all caffeine must be eliminated,* even that morning cup of coffee. This step is *absolutely essential and mandatory.* If the patient must have coffee, it must be decaffeinated.

The other general sleep guidelines Joe followed are as follows:

a. Wind down before bedtime. Do not pay bills or make stressful phone calls within several hours of going to bed.
b. Don't eat a large meal just prior to going to bed, as this will interfere with a restful night's sleep. Eat a sensible dinner at least three or four hours before bedtime and then avoid late-night snacking.
c. Follow a regular time schedule for going to bed and waking up. Stick with the schedule as rigidly as possible.
d. Develop a relaxing routine immediately before bedtime. Some people relax by reading or watching TV.
e. While exercising during the day may help you sleep better at night, do not exercise too close to bedtime, as this will interfere with winding down.

f. Make your bed, your nighttime attire, and the temperature in your room comfortable.

g. Make sure the place where you sleep is quiet.

h. Do not have a desk or business phone in the bedroom. Make your bedroom a place that is primarily for sleeping.

i. Avoid having heavy conversations with family members or others just prior to going to bed. Unless it is an emergency, that kind of talk can usually be put off until morning.

j. Do not drink alcohol within three or four hours of bedtime. Of course, excessive alcohol consumption at any time, a problem in itself, will only compound both sleep and interpersonal difficulties and therefore must be dealt with before attempting to address any sleep problem.

Joe had been violating some of these commonsense sleep recommendations, but he made adjustments in order to at least provide the framework for a restful night's sleep. Adhering to these guidelines was relatively easy.

Step 2

At my suggestion, Joe began this crucial step by further exploring his new understandings about his childhood dysfunction and abuse with a qualified therapist. When I shared with him the latest findings, which confirmed a concrete link between his abusive past and his lifelong Type B Night Terror problem, something his new therapist had long suspected anyway, his past trauma was validated and his therapy became even more focused and productive.

Some have written about the dire consequences of failing to recognize and treat past trauma. Others have reported the positive outcome of intervention that begins by dealing with that trauma. In studying night terrors almost forty years ago, Leopold and Dillon wrote: "Psychological damage incurred in life-threatening trauma, if untreated, tends to grow worse with time." (16, pp.919, 920)

Regarding untreated psychological damage of the severity which could lead to Type B Night Terrors, Carol Glod wrote: "It is conceivable that early intervention targeted at abused children with sleep disruption may help diminish long-term intractable insomnia. Adults with a history of early childhood trauma frequently report persistent disruptions in sleep that may be relatively refractory to treatment. Early intervention may be of value in mitigating this potentially enduring effect." (10, p.1243) And early intervention appears to have been effective in treating the victims of the Chowchilla, California, kidnapping. Susan Knapp reported that: "Some of the children, however, continued to have night terror episodes until they received psychotherapy which dealt with the kidnapping." (5, p.193)

Also, out of necessity, Joe severed many dysfunctional family ties. This is similar to what Munchausen by proxy syndrome victim Mary Bryk had done. She explained her reasons when she wrote: "I invited my parents, brother and sister to meet with me and my therapist. My brother, with whom I'm only intermittently in touch, chose not to come. I confronted my family directly, telling them my mother had deliberately abused me as a child; she fit the profile of Munchausen by proxy syndrome, I said, handing them articles on the subject. I wasn't surprised when she denied everything, nor that my father and sister believed her and not me. My mother is a very intelligent, very manipulative person who can be extremely convincing, and my father and sister had always wanted to believe her, no matter what. The only contact I've had with my family since then was a letter from my sister telling me that she no longer wanted any contact with me." (52, p.96)

As in Mary's case, many family members may side with the abuser. Maintaining contact with such individuals is not only empty and unfulfilling but also extremely stressful and damaging. Severing or limiting such empty and/or harmful ties is difficult. Dr. Chu explained that those who have been exposed to severe trauma may seek to distance themselves from their devastating experiences either by "emotional denial" or by bonding with their "idealized caretakers," who are often the very persons responsible for abusing them. (34, p.82)

Joe's comprehension of the magnitude of dysfunction in his childhood home only became clear to him through envisioning his own children suffering what he suffered. This led him to understand the discomfort he had always felt when talking to his parents. While others may or may not feel compelled to sever these types of dysfunctional relations, Joe felt he had to do so for his own good. Nothing about his parents had improved or changed. They remained exactly as they always had been.

While many people, including therapists, have strong opinions about the severing of blood ties, only the abused person is qualified to decide what is right for his or her own life. No one else has walked in his or her shoes, and few people can even relate to some of the things that may be in the abuse victim's past. Such was the case with Nancy, one of Dr. Chu's patients. In describing her experiences, he pointed out that Nancy had nothing but contempt for her mother and for her alcoholic and psychotic father. According to her own accounts during treatment, her father had inflicted brutal and near murderous abuse upon her, including throwing her out of a window, which resulted in fractures of her arm, ribs, and skull that could still be traced through radiology. (34, p.198)

Is it healthy for Nancy to remain in contact with such parents? Many judgmental people base their uninformed opinion about these types of decisions on their own interaction with relatively normal and loving parents, with whom they were fortunate enough to grow up. They fail to realize that "parent" is not a universal constant. But, as with all abuse victims, Nancy would be the only one fully qualified to evaluate whether or not to continue associating with her parents.

This decision cannot be made with any degree of reliability until the victim has worked through all forms of denial and suppression of the abuse and faced the reality of his or her past honestly and openly. Therefore, although the severing of all involvement with his abusers was one of the first steps that Joe took in dealing directly with his night terror problem, he had spent years coming to terms with and even confronting his parents about the abuse they had perpetrated on him. He did not sever his relationship with them to avoid the challenging work he had to do; he severed the relationship only after painstakingly working through these deep, difficult, and oftentimes confrontational issues. Some individuals may decide not to sever ties with their abusers, depending on their own circumstances and the nature of their present interactions with the abusers. But the decision must always be theirs to make.

Step 3

At the same time Joe was addressing his past through therapy, he was also learning a great deal about his present circumstances, both in therapy and on his own. After identifying Lucy as a rage-a-holic who was also incapable of either speaking truthfully or trusting others, there was plenty of pertinent and relevant information to be found. He came to understand the motivations behind all of Lucy's actions and learned how to avoid setting her off. He stopped trying to communicate with her in the open, honest, sincere fashion with which he communicated with his children and friends.

Conversation with someone who is filled with pain and cannot trust others serves little purpose. No intimacy is going to grow, no closeness is going to result, and no relationship is going to be built. Magid and McKelvy reported that people like Lucy are far less angry and volatile toward individuals who *"don't try to develop a close, caring reciprocal relationship."* (38, p.56) This is partially why Lucy had always gravitated toward one-night stands with old boyfriends and sexual interactions with strangers she met in bars. She had a lifelong pattern of only being comfortable in superficial, empty interpersonal encounters.

Joe now listened to Lucy, agreed with her, and refrained from commenting on any of her lies or self-delusions. He stayed away from any subject that was deep, truthful, or intimate. Speaking from the heart to an individual who has no interest in any form of interpersonal, personal, or spiritual growth is pointless. All words and actions emanating from Joe or anyone else were filtered and distorted by the ill will, suspicion, defensiveness, and deep mistrust within which Lucy had entombed herself for her entire life. Joe came to understand that only Lucy could free herself from this prison. Cracking open this closed, wave-pounded shell was not his job. He basically conformed to what Lucy had wanted from the beginning: to be left alone with her emptiness, secrets, and lies while pretending to be involved in a marriage. Interestingly, Lucy started seeing herself as a person who had dramatically matured and mellowed, unaware that it was Joe making all the adjustments.

In a more affirmative move, Joe imposed boundaries and limits on Lucy. He came to realize that the only thing that stood between Lucy and adultery was opportunity. He set limits on the places that she could be and the people that she could be with. He made it clear that in spite of the lack of boundaries in the family in which she was raised, her habit of promiscuity, and the rampant sexual affairs of almost everyone she knew, he would no longer tolerate such behavior on her part. Joe did not bother to explain the true meaning of marriage, fidelity, and appropriate sexual expression. Lucy was incapable of comprehending anything about those concepts. Besides, everything about her understanding of sexuality was awry. Dr. Chu wrote that people such as Lucy, with a history of childhood sexual abuse, are so disoriented that they "even invite the therapist to engage in sexual relationships," and "are more likely to be the victims of therapists' sexual misconduct." (34, pp.133, 103)

However, Joe did explain to her that adultery makes promises it can't keep. After the act is consummated, few people feel better about themselves, only cheap, dirty, and used. He pointed out that if adultery could satisfy, Lucy would have been fully satisfied by now. She was then given the choice of accepting monogamy and its limits, or leaving. It was made clear to her that having it both ways would no longer be acceptable. If bed-hopping was how she wanted to live out the rest of her life, then she would have to remove Joe's bed from her list!

While everything about this situation would probably be un-workable for an emotionally normal person, Joe wasn't in that category. A tenuous peace ensued precisely because this entire scenario was very familiar. Joe had spent his entire childhood ap-peasing hateful, abusive people. Once he understood who and what Lucy was, getting along with her became relatively easy.

Step 4

Joe also began addressing his night terror and stress-related health problems. He found the information that I showed him about the link between extreme trauma, Type B Night Terrors, and later health problems to be both fascinating and pertinent. During his marriage to Lucy, he had not only been experiencing an inordinate number of colds but had developed eczema and was almost con-tinually battling skin rashes on various parts of his body.

After dealing with his past and present emotional problems and seeing a dramatic drop-off in his night terror symptoms, he also noticed the almost complete disappearance of his eczema and skin rashes. The many over-the-counter and prescription ointments and medications that Joe had used on his skin during his entire marriage were no longer necessary. The only residual effects were some skin discoloration and several patches of wrin-kled and damaged skin. (These effects were the result of years of using increasingly potent topical medications to try to control the skin rashes and eczema.) In ultimately solving his skin problem, Joe realized that no amount or strength of medication or ointment would have eliminated the rashes, since they were a byproduct of the emotional stress in his life and his night terror disturbed sleep.

Step 5

Joe was a very responsible person—probably too responsible. His attention to detail and perfection in everything he did suggests that he may have had some obsessive/compulsive tendencies. As a result, his schedule was always full and he was busy from morning till night. His commitment to his job, family, and home left Joe little time for himself. Therefore, he did something that was extremely important for his own healing. Joe began to allow himself at least two hours of solitude per day. It would have made no sense for him to have bombarded himself with explosive childhood emotional issues and then not allow himself time during the day to attempt to sort out and come to terms with all this weighty information. It would have been counterproductive to rip open all these emotional wounds and then not grant himself a little daily recuperation or recovery time. It might have become overwhelming to ingest all this intense stress without giving himself a daily stress-releasing outlet.

Joe scheduled at least one hour a day for walking along the beach, park, or other tranquil setting and just thinking. He would have taken more time for his walks if he had felt he needed it. For the first time in years he wasn't checking his watch. Daily reading time was also allowed, in which he would investigate literature on childhood trauma, relationships, or whatever he felt a need to learn more about. He also allowed himself time every day to exercise in order to allay or channel his stress into physical activity.

Daily physical activity, including at least a short period of vigorous exercise, is an essential outlet for very passive people like Joe. Like other night terror sufferers, his peaceful, nonconfrontational demeanor, inability to react to any affront, inappropriately excessive self-control, and strict moral, overly civil and/or religiously motivated behavioral self-constraints afforded him virtually no other outlet for pent-up anxiety or stress. In contrast to those people who act out their lifelong pain on others, Joe, who rarely acted on internal feelings or external pressures, needed the emotionally liberating benefits of physical activity and exercise. He also made a point of taking a short twenty-minute nap each afternoon. Joe would sleep at his desk, in his car, or wherever he happened to be. As noted in the professional literature, such short daily naps have very real benefits for both Type A and Type B night terror sufferers.

Joe didn't explain or confer with anybody in his family about his decisions. He knew what he needed. If he had been trying to recover from numerous serious physical injuries, he would have allowed himself the time to recover. Just about everyone would have been able to understand because most physical maladies are obvious to the observer. Joe saw himself as trying to recover from numerous serious emotional injuries, which were very difficult for most people to understand. Therefore, he no longer allowed himself to care what other people thought. He came to see and understand the true seriousness of his emotional injuries. Without allowing himself special time for recovery, it's doubtful that his attempts at making connections, mastering stresses, learning new coping behaviors and adaptations, and lessening the frequency of his night terror symptoms would have been as successful as it eventually was. Therefore, allowing himself special recovery times on a daily basis was an absolutely essential step. No night terror sufferer or therapist should overlook or minimize this crucial requirement.

Step 6

Progress in the five steps above came relatively easily. Although Joe instituted the five steps in the order listed above, in a short while he was engaged in implementing all the stages simultaneously. This constitutes the sixth step.

Many professional books on psychotherapy divide the treatment course into early, middle, and late stages. The earliest stage deals with developing a positive self-image and practical relational skills. The middle stage usually involves confronting and addressing the victim's traumatic past in an open and straightforward manner. The last stage deals with reinforcing the new understandings and applying them to the real world.

Because Type B Night Terror sufferers are mostly functional, trusting, forward-moving individuals, the first two stages progress quickly with very little resistance. Typically, these people have been overcoming obstacles for their entire lives. Most of them know that they have the power to change things and to grow. Perseverance and conquering challenges have been a way of life for them. Therefore, they are likely to be good candidates for effective therapeutic intervention.

Type B Night Terror sufferers are not chronically disempowered; they are just the opposite. The chronically disempowered routinely avoid all light-shedding and truth-shedding processes, of which therapy is one of the highest forms. Therefore, they usually avoid therapy. But even if forced into it, they distrust the therapist and therefore rely on the manipulation and lies that have been the foundation of their entire lives. In all the case studies I've read about that deal with these kinds of people, therapists spent years simply trying to get these chronically disempowered persons to be real and truthful. Usually this attempt has failed. And while the therapist was trying to convince the patient to take some responsibility and begin to play a role in his or her own healing and improvement, that person was playing games, trying to get the therapist to be totally responsible for whatever might happen.

Dr. Chu explained that patients with a sufficient sense of "self-empowerment" will try to emulate the support, validation, and caring that the therapist provides for them. Those who are chronically disempowered will only see the therapist's actions as substitutes for their own efforts to develop those same qualities, and will constantly seek to have him or her do more for them. (34, p.191)

Type B Night Terror sufferers are characteristically very hard-working when it comes to striving after and achieving goals. Throughout life, things that normal people take for granted have typically required a huge amount of effort for the Type B Night Terror sufferer. Many of these sufferers have become somewhat functional because of their work ethic and because of their usual lack of fear when presented with challenges. This is another off-shoot of the gradual changes in perspective that a Type B Night Terror sufferer goes through.

Most of the night terror victims I've encountered are confident that they can do anything they put their minds to and are willing to work at. Success in overcoming obstacles breeds self-confidence. And the night terror victim's entire life has been a never-ending succession of hurdles and obstacles to be overcome.

On the other hand, the Lucys of this world have given up a long time ago. They have usually turned into manipulative abusers themselves. These people sleep very well; they're not holding anything in. They are acting out their hate and lifelong rage on others; there's little for them to deal with at night. Interestingly, when the chronically disempowered are forced to confront some truth about themselves in therapy, they often begin to experience minor sleep disruption.

Fortunately, it is characteristic of many Type B Night Terror victims that they already possess all the internal tools to make productive therapy possible. Dr. Chu indicated that patients who have the best chance of attaining a normal life after severe trauma are those who are willing to make the necessary effort by taking charge of their own lives, and willing to look at obstacles as challenges rather than roadblocks. (34, p.77) These traits have been the essence of the Type B Night Terror victim's entire life.

Dr. Chu has revealed what probably happened to Joe in his healing process. He wrote: "They become more skilled in dealing with their lives. [This is because of] having been able to acknowledge their past traumatization and having found ways to engage others despite having been victimized." (34, pp.207, 208) The bottom line is that the successful end product which all Type B Night Terror sufferers seek must of necessity be the result of a great deal of painful effort and hard work.

Finally, one of Dr. Chu's patients summed up exactly how I myself view the journey that led to my own Type B Night Terror cure and also resulted in the writing of this book: *I now know that I'm a good and decent person. I like myself and other people, and I know how to deal with the world—perhaps even better than people who haven't had to go through what I've gone through. I not only exist in life, but I actually live my life."* (34, p.208)

)

PART TWO

A THERAPIST'S GUIDANCE

by Jane R. Dill, Ph.D., L.M.F.T., D.A.P.A.

Chapter 14

Exploring Trauma and Its Effects

In a dark time, the eye begins to see.
—Theodore Roethke

A New Awareness

For the most part, we Americans lived in a "happiness culture" before 9/11. It had been a long time since there was war on our own soil. Generally protected by military might, two oceans, and victory, our culture centered on upward mobility and the good life. I used to hear from clients that all they wanted was to be happy, which to them meant repressing anything negative—a form of denial. Happiness is a wonderful thing if it doesn't gloss over the realities of life within the family as well as the community, nation, and world. But the terrorism of 9/11 has brought the horrors of war home to all Americans. Individually and collectively we have been steeped in fear, pain, anxiety, and anger.

Since September 11, 2001, many brochures from national seminar organizations arriving at my private office proffer the latest techniques for treating trauma. It often takes a national crisis to highlight a relatively neglected area of concern. Though over the last twenty years trauma has been recognized in sexual and physical abuse victims, war veterans, and Holocaust victims, professionals and laypersons alike continue to struggle with finding effective solutions to many of its consequences, such as memory formation, memory recall, dissociation, recurring nightmares, night terrors, neglect, and emotional abuse. Even in the current crescendo of trauma information, the effect of a single incident takes center stage, covering over the complexity and depth of the overall topic of trauma as well as its effect on victims.

As mentioned earlier in the book, in the past the connection between extreme trauma and the subsequent development of nightmares, night terrors, and other psychological aberrations among survivors has been questioned because there has been a great time differential between cause and effect. The short time frame between 9/11 and the emergence of severe nightmares and/or night terrors corroborates the definitive link between trauma and such symptoms. Chronic forms of these disorders reported among 350 New York firefighters present a unique group scenario in the field of trauma study. It's likely that this particular report, less than six months after the event, is only the tip of the iceberg.

The complexity of night terrors has been uncovered by Mr. Carranza's pertinent research. To unravel the web of trauma we must consider a continuum of extreme trauma and terror. At one end is the simplicity of a direct connection between an event or incident experienced by a child who was frightened by a shadow. At the opposite end of the continuum is the chronic, long-term terror of a child's or an adult's Holocaust, both of whom survive with permanent scars. The treatment of such human experiences needs to take into account the duration and the many varying degrees of trauma that exist.

Both the short-term and long-term effects of trauma have been and still are seen simply as something the sufferer has to get over. The subject of pain and death itself has often been avoided. As early as the 1960s there was so much denial regarding death that Dr. Elizabeth Kübler-Ross's book on *Death and Dying* seemed more shocking than death itself. Some titles on the subject even suggested that death had to come "out of the closet." Grieving, a natural process after trauma for all humans around the world, remains largely misunderstood and suppressed in some Western countries, including the United States. Therefore, promoting and helping along the grieving process has become a standard specialty in therapeutic practices. Our culture's denial of the validity of pain and grieving as part of the healing process delays recovery.

We are in a new cultural environment since 9/11 and since the recent increase in school shootings. Everyone in the United States has become painfully aware of our vulnerability and the aftermath of trauma. We can no longer deny that terror can hit us in our "safe places." Our schools are no longer safe from terror. Our land, formerly protected by oceans and missiles, is no longer safe. Nor are our homes. We can no longer see ourselves as invincible.

Trauma-related nightmares and night terrors are now exposed, reported in the newspapers as affecting New York firefighters and school children. But what surprised me was that three professional seminars on trauma and terrorism in the year 2002 mentioned neither nightmares nor night terrors as symptoms. One conference included eight international experts, two of whom, when asked directly, said they didn't know anything about night terrors. Nor were trauma-related nightmares mentioned in their extensive lists of symptoms. In another seminar an internationally known expert on crisis intervention would not take a few moments to talk to me about night terrors, but he said he had seen many people with them. He never mentioned trauma-related nightmares during the seminar. At another seminar I asked a psychologist, an evaluator for the courts who determines placement for convicted criminals, if she had come across reports of night terrors and trauma-related nightmares in this highly traumatized population. Indeed, she had seen many such cases but had seen no related materials.

However, there is and always has been hope. Hope is found in reality and knowledge, not in fantasy and ignorance. Raising the awareness of and establishing the existence of night terrors force us also to examine the subject of trauma-related nightmares. Before significant research into the brain, trauma-related nightmares were considered the intrusion of evil or representations of the devil. Some dream interpreters and laypersons still believe this to be true. Others believe dreams and nightmares to be a trick of the mind and that the best results come by dismissing them or even by having the patient take sleep medication to overcome them. These kinds of responses leave nightmare and night terror sufferers with the impression that they are the problem, rather than being the victims of trauma.

At this juncture in current thinking, it becomes valuable to develop practical and realistic ways to describe how nightmares and night terrors relate to our daily lives and how this knowledge can enhance our understanding of ourselves and our ability to deal with trauma and terror. Our first job is to understand how being asleep and being awake relate. Because of the early pioneers in psychology such as Freud and Jung, we have perceived the sleep world as the unconscious, a kind of mystical place where our worst self resides. Freud's emphasis on sexual interpretations of dreams and Jung's emphasis on representational archetypes from the collective unconscious have produced helpful and enjoyable interpretations. However, because of neurobiopsychological study of the brain in the last twenty years, we can add a scientific view of dreams, nightmares, and night terrors.

In the spirit of new discoveries about the brain and its functions, in particular those regarding memory, I wish to help point out that symptoms from the ravages of severe trauma can be overcome. Rather than call the hidden, sleep functioning of the brain the unconscious, I am going to refer to it as sleep thinking. When I refer to the general term trauma-related nightmares I shall be including nightmares that are caused by either single- or multi-incident traumas. The term nightmares will include all the kinds of nightmares. These do not include night terrors, which are completely different from nightmares.

Primary and Secondary Trauma

Trauma is defined as severe, intense, sharp, overwhelming fear in the face of danger. It may come from a single crisis, Trauma I, or ongoing multi-incident terror over a period of time, Trauma II. Trauma creates shock from a startling experience with a lasting effect. Put these together and we have the foundation for severe psychological damage. Trauma, but especially extreme trauma and terror, challenges everything we believe about ourselves, others, relationships, humanity, God. Our ideals are broken at the same time we cling to them. We begin living in the extremes. Or perhaps we have been in the life of extremes and the trauma reinforced them. Our values are challenged. Our needs are frozen in time. The meaning of life is confronted. Our unexamined life is frozen until it gets in our way years later. Even the event is distorted. Each trauma has its own meaning to the individual. "Meanings depend upon ethnic, religious, familial and personal contributions, along with residues from previous traumas." (55, p.11)

Smucker and Dancu describe a Type 1 Trauma and a Type 2 Trauma. Type 1 is unexpected and isolated, as was 9/11. This is the single-incident trauma that comes from earthquakes and other natural disasters. It often involves many people who can commiserate with each other about their experience and loss.

Type 2 trauma is expected and chronic. These traumas often lead to personality disorders, patterns of defense mechanisms, self-abuse and the abuse of others, threats, and attempts at suicide. The symptoms include recurrence of traumatic memories in trauma-related nightmares and night terrors. In these cases the responses to the trauma become the concern. The result of centering one's life on survival creates denial, inadequacy, helplessness, abandonment, and recurring sleeping or waking memories that re-traumatize the individual. This is unfinished business that needs to be dealt with before it propagates and festers. Even those who are trained to do crisis intervention are not protected from the symptoms of post-traumatic stress disorder (PTSD). Vulnerable to what has been labeled "secondary trauma," caretakers, though not directly suffering from a traumatic event, are exposed to horrific stories and/or injuries. If they rationalize that they cannot eat, sleep, or take time out, they also become victims with PTSD symptoms. Such symptoms may be called burnout or compassion fatigue.

The traumas of single events like 9/11 or random shootings are difficult, even if the individual is accustomed to catastrophe. Firemen see tragedy and loss of life, but it is hard to cope with people jumping from windows to save themselves from a vicious attack that seems to make no sense. It is hard to know that you are helpless to save those you are trained to save, including your fellow firefighters. In such tragedies feelings are often set aside to perform a duty. Obviously our memories have been affected. The New York firefighters had nightmares and night terrors. I am certain more segments of the population not directly involved also developed these kinds of symptoms. Sleep disruption should push those secondary victims to look at the real experience, share it with those who are supportive, get rid of any untruths, and work out ways to cope with any other trauma that may come along. This process of debriefing is essential for emotional health and will be explained in detail in the next chapter.

One trauma victim often misunderstood and neglected is that secondary trauma sufferer. Secondary trauma happens to those who are on the sidelines of the terror. The traumatic event does not happen directly to the individual adult or child. The effects of secondary trauma are evidenced in the study mentioned earlier which indicated that 90 percent of New York City school children were suffering at least one symptom of post-traumatic stress disorder related to the 9/11 terror attacks. Additionally, although none of these children were at ground zero, over 40 percent reported sleeping problems or nightmares. Secondary trauma symptoms such as burnout or compassion fatigue were evidenced by many caregivers who worked closely with those who were directly traumatized.

Due to the urgency of the situation, caregivers often refuse to take necessary rests, meals, and sleep that could refurbish the mental, emotional, and physical energy needed to truly help the victims. It may be evident that helpers, like the victims, are re-traumatized by repetitive telling of victims' stories. Everyone involved in any kind of trauma needs to be aware of the need for relief from the trauma. That relief comes more quickly if, within the first three months after the incident, the victim gets a chance in a safe place to debrief by talking it through with a compassionate, supportive person. Telling someone merely to "get on with your life" is neither compassionate nor supportive. These kinds of responses to another's pain and fear negate feelings and prolong the agony.

Now the event that caused the trauma, repressed and defended, is remembered in fragments and buried feelings. The mind tries to make sense of this incomplete distorted picture. "Traumatic events are processed in terms of a victim's emotional stability and pre-traumatic ways of taking up reality. Interpersonal support, along with ethnic and religious ways of making sense, influence whether or not victims will be able to contain and eventually grow from new learning generated by their traumatic experiences." (55, p.15)

Sleep Thinking

Nightmares vary in content and relate to the dreamer's current life events or feelings. Remember that nightmares do refer in some way to a perceived or real trauma in our life. The triggering trauma, though unsettling for the dreamer, is transitory. In her book *In Your Dreams,* Gayle Delaney clearly reminds us that our dreams are individual; we create them. She cautions us that other people's ideas of what our dreams might mean are not necessarily our own meaning. Dream experts believe that sleep thinking is an attempt of the mind to make connections, to resolve something, or to find the place to store it in memory. Barrett wrote: "Many creative and problem-solving dreams are nightmares. Our dream ego is just not concerned with the original problem—but some other part of us is. It grabs our attention with any means at its disposal." (56, p.170)

We might consider sleep thinking as a kind of meditation that the mind is doing to fulfill its function. In meditation we try to shut out any assault on our consciousness. We have no need to move. We are free to be with our thoughts and free from caring about our environment and those in it. We are simply with ourselves. What is left are images and encoded reactions. As in meditation or daydreaming, sometimes an image or feeling pushes through to dreams during sleep.

Studies shed light on these processes. Barrett reported on a study of multiple personality dreamers. "[The] personalities showed up as dream characters giving the host advice or offering information about the past." (56, pp.186–187) Any beginning psychology student remembering the split-brain studies will recall that when the two brain hemispheres were surgically separated the nonverbal side could still direct the conscious mind through touch. The brain is not one cohesive unit but different sections that must make connections to be whole. If we don't make the necessary connections or something isn't resolved, the brain will let us know through feelings, nightmares, night terrors, or patterns of behavior that something needs to be dealt with. Dr. Daniel Amen's studies of spectrometer brain scans dramatically and in vivid color show all the areas where feelings such as anger reside. The brain is always processing.

"The major concerns of dreaming are obviously our personal issues: childhood slights, current moods, and how we get along with significant others." (56, p.ix) During dreams our brains are free to give our minds an opportunity to express our feelings—anger, hurt, fear and anxiety. Delaney wrote, "When we sleep we do some of our most creative, least defensive, and most insightful thinking. . . . You use images and themes drawn from your life experience to make metaphors or parables that express how you really feel and what you really think about your life as seen from your sleeping mind's perspective." (57 p.5)

When nightmares recur repeatedly over time, it is as if the sleep thinking mind wants something solved, something resolved. The stored images and feelings freed from consciousness by sleep haven't found a place in memory that connects them. The memory is still active. Such memories need to be divested of feeling energy or dealt with sufficiently enough to be "filed" or released. The mind in sleep now opens to consider what the conscious mind has repressed, pushed aside, and attempted to cover up.

While sleep thinking continues to work on our problems, the nightmare or night terror symptoms are disturbing our lives. Parents or significant others report the victim's symptoms but do not know the causes. Nightmares and night terrors keep partners, as well as sufferers, concerned. Consequently, the underlying problems can fester for years until other behavioral symptoms arise. Because these symptoms are not rational but representational, the realization that there are real connections to be made may not surface until the sufferer gets into a close relationship. Most of my clients with recurring nightmares or other sleep disorders came to therapy to solve relationship problems. One couple was even concerned about bringing a child into the world of such disturbing symptoms.

The Memory Process

Nightmares and other sleep disorders can happen to anyone. Why is it that, in both perceived and real crises, some people develop nightmares and some don't? A number of determiners have been identified.

First, the age of the person experiencing the incident(s) highlights developmental considerations such as brain growth and psychosocial tasks. A child whose brain networks have not sufficiently developed to understand either the elements of a trauma or its significance may compartmentalize the parts he/she perceives or fears. This can lead to dissociation, a fragmenting of elements into memory. An older child or an adult might apply his/her own interpretation to an incident trying to establish some sense, in order to avoid thinking of it because it is too fearful to see as it is. "Laughing away one's own suffering is a form of fending off pain, a response that can prevent us from seeing and tapping the sources of understanding around us." (58, p. 105)

Second, the length of time the trauma is endured determines if the victim has developed behavioral patterns and mental networks that protect him/her from the effects of abuse. If a child or adult is confronted with a traumatic incident and has developed coping skills, those abilities will help debrief the terror and allow the individual to face it realistically. If the person has not learned coping techniques while attending to life's traumas, his or her chances of having trauma-related nightmares increase exponentially. Once a trauma has been experienced and filed in memory without debriefing, it will continue to affect the reaction to traumas that follow.

Third, reports of children and adults who are very intelligent and creative and who have faced frightening events suggest that such people are most susceptible to nightmares and other sleep disorders. They tend to be hypersensitive to their environment and have vivid imaging capabilities. This mental and sensory agility expedites the encoding of images and feelings that seem to enrich their dream or nightmare world.

Fourth, infancy and preverbal experiences with chronic abuse or chronic anxiety are reported to last a lifetime. This and any chemical imbalance might lead to multiple disorders. Traumas, added to other personality disorders, create additional difficulties for victims and those around them. Many personality disorders begin with traumas. Trauma-related nightmares can signal such disorders.

The brain keeps active whether we pay attention or not. Dreams, particularly nightmares, are capable of waking us up in the middle of the night, suddenly causing us to remember something we had been concerned about. Artists, writers, and scientists often speak of waking up with solutions to problems in their work. Perhaps we are angry and we haven't taken care of a problem. Maybe we don't remember abuse by someone but we instinctively withdraw from that person. The brain keeps trying to make sense of it, to make connections until we consciously "get it."

I share with clients what is essential for them to understand. It is that the brain continues to think or actively make connections and store information while we sleep. If the brain stops processing thoughts and information, we are dead. Electroencepholographs (EEGs) of brain activity show that we have high spiking graph lines (beta) for high energy levels; lower, broader spiking graph lines (alpha) for general brain energy; shorter and broader theta spikes for drowsiness; and short and even broader spikes for delta sleep. When the brain is no longer processing information, the line is flat and we are brain dead. The conclusion can only be that if any brain energy remains, we are in some ways still thinking during sleep, probably by rearranging and adding to our memories. "Neurology suggests that dreaming is simply the mind thinking in a different biochemical mode." (56, p.184)

Another critical aspect of the memory process is the role of perception. When awake, we believe that we are processing whatever is happening to us. Critically, our senses may take in or filter out much of the information we think we have perceived. A classic sociology study found that college students would walk right by an actor who was stumbling and swaying if they thought the man was drunk. If they thought the man was having a heart attack, they would stop to help him. How many times do we drive past a disabled car at the side of the road and rationalize that the driver must have a cell phone, that he/she is just resting, or that if we stop we might find ourselves in trouble? Our perceptions and rationalizations overcome the moment of stress; we let it go and soon forget the situation. Thus, our memory may be faulty, though we believe it to be true. If we have strong hidden feelings such as guilt or fear, trauma-related nightmares may be the result.

Sometimes fear causes us to perceive narrowly what is happening because we need to concentrate on surviving. Thus, a bystander not so threatened may remember the scene more accurately, yet we may still be certain he/she is wrong. Couples spend hours arguing about his perception versus her perception over a past event. Each remembers only that which angered or hurt him or her. Many don't even remember what they were arguing over but remain upset. Each person focused on only one phrase that hurt, did not hear the rest, and now insists that what he/she remembers is wholly accurate.

So, at times, information or thoughts do not get past short-term memory into long-term. We rationalize, repress, misperceive, or simply take in only parts or fragments of a given event. I'm certain all persons have had some great thoughts only to be unable to remember what they were. They had them but didn't do anything with them. In the relationship with ourselves as well as with others, in order to remember we must attach energy through doing as well as feeling or thinking.

Talking about something is a form of practice which helps one remember. Debriefing is a way to connect information received so as to recreate the reality of a given event. Writing ideas down helps implant thoughts and information into the brain memory or the muscle memory. If you practice a baseball swing or the swing of a tennis racket, the steps of a dance, a piece on the piano, or the ABC song, the activity becomes a habit memory.

An incorrect or partly incorrect memory not challenged at the time imbeds the information and cheats us of a fuller understanding of any incident or robs us of healing. If a child sees a violent television program, becomes fearful and refuses to go to sleep afterwards, and if the parent gets angry at him/her for not obeying, that parent has not validated the fact that the child has a right to feelings. Nor has the parent helped the child to understand that the show was made of pictures and would not happen while he/she was asleep. Sometimes adults forget that kids don't know what adults know. As a result, the child may begin to form a pattern of not showing feelings to the parent. Their relationship is then damaged. Over time, the continual practice of not showing feelings can become a pattern which may feed nightmares or other sleep disturbances.

Patterns are formed from beliefs. Let's call the abovementioned child Teddy. He believes that something he saw on television can happen to him. His parents have forgotten how scared they could be as children, and they are tired. Not wanting to take a few minutes to help Teddy cope with his fears, they send the signal that he is the problem. He is causing them trouble. If this occurs in other areas of Teddy's life, he believes he is the trouble and that he is wrong to have feelings. He may become quiet or may act out his trouble. This pattern of not speaking feelings may lose him his marriage and even his job years later. Most of my private practice consists of helping clients as old as sixty to recognize such patterns and providing help if they want to change them. Understanding the purpose of feelings, customs, beliefs, faith, process, memory, possibilities, and goals is vital to understanding trauma, nightmares, and other sleep disorders, and vice versa.

A Case History

Robert (a composite of several clients) was forty-eight years old when he came to my office because his wife and children were leaving him. Both Robert and Marian were successful upper middle class professionals. Marian's major complaint was Robert's unwillingness to discuss anything. This left all the decisions up to her. The few times he did get upset, he raged. Interestingly enough, Robert taught communication at the local community college and helped businesses by giving seminars on better interpersonal relationships. His three children ranged from six to twenty, the oldest going to college while still living at home.

In his own defense, Robert felt that Marian was like his mother, a critical woman who had two other children with serious illnesses. While he was growing up, his mother simply couldn't stop caretaking long enough to sympathize with him. He was the youngest of three in his family. His alcoholic father worked full-time plus overtime, and when he came home he ate, drank, watched television, and yelled at Robert. As a boy, Robert early adopted the pattern of getting out of the way, not causing his parents to get upset, and doing things on his own. All his life he considered himself the ultimate problem solver. Marian was not interested in couple therapy because they had been in therapy before and it hadn't worked. Though Robert felt feelings and tried to hide them, he admitted that Marian could tell when he was feeling angry or down.

The Importance of Feelings

"When feelings speak, we are compelled to listen—and sometimes act—even if we do not always understand why. Not to be aware of one's feelings, not to understand them or know how to use or express them, is worse than being blind, deaf or paralyzed." (59, p.9) If we let the moment go by, we may well get off the track by hearing something other than the real meaning or the immediate concern.

As suggested earlier, feelings have a valid place in our lives. If denied, we lose major opportunities for relating. When I ask clients how they show emotional hurt, they often refer to crying over the death of a significant other. I ask them what they do when they feel not listened to or are disrespected. They indicate that they say nothing or become angry. When asked what they do when they are scared, they indicate they frequently deny being afraid, get angry, or don't say anything. When angered many yell, withdraw, throw things, or get sarcastic. Such patterns were developed in childhood.

Robert told me that his father yelled, threatened, and shoved, while his mother kept her feelings inside. Our initial session was the first time that he had made the connection between his own behavior and that of his parents. He hadn't believed his wife when she said his problems stemmed from his childhood.

Then he told me about his recurring nightmares that began at age four. They became less frequent as he aged but occurred whenever he was under stress. Until he was fourteen his mother told him he would sit up in bed, scream, and push away anyone who got near. The nightmares happened off and on about once a month. Robert's parents scolded him for waking them up at all hours of the night. He didn't know what they were talking about until his mother took him with one of his sick siblings to the doctor. The physician told her Robert was having nightmares and that they would go away in time. They never went away, and when 9/11 occurred, his nightmares became more frequent, intense, and chronic.

Too often we do not consider the effects of trauma on the family and particularly on siblings with mental and physical illnesses and addictions. Some professionals forget to consider the effect a sufferer has on the entire family structure. When a person presents a problem like trauma-related nightmares, it may be treated by the family as an individual sickness, so other family members ignore the effect on them.

In Robert's case, sympathy seemed to go mostly to the sick children and the caretaking mother. Robert looked like a well-adapted child by comparison. He was so busy in childhood and adulthood defending his feelings and beliefs about incidents in his life that they became embedded in memory. His sleep thinking pulled up feelings and symbols into nightmares, telling him that something important in his life needed to be dealt with.

The first advice of most dream experts is to identify the feeling(s) of the nightmare sufferer. There is good reason for this. Our feelings are one of the first indications that we have of trouble. We see, hear, smell, touch, taste then feel physical or emotional pain. The body flashes warnings. Unfortunately, when we have grown up in a culture or family that denies pain or believes that feeling pain is wimpish, we drown out these warnings and suppress them under denial, anger, superiority, and many other defense mechanisms. We hide in false happiness or become bitter because life isn't as the American Dream promised. Even after seeing violent or depressing movies, many of us walk away saying, My life isn't that bad by comparison; I can minimize my troubles. But sleep thinking warns us to face up, not minimize. It tells us to deal with all problems when they arise, or suffer the consequences.

The mind requires a threshold of feeling intense enough to get our attention. We don't remember the commonplace, the routine. Indeed, habits that no longer require attention simply seem to happen automatically. Robert presented an example of this phenomenon when he told me in the first session that he experienced anger and hurt in his head. He freely admitted he did not know when these feelings were occurring; he just reacted. Not feeling his feelings and now not speaking his feelings had damaged his marriage. In a sudden realization, Robert admitted he could see how this habit corrupted his relationship with co-workers, particularly his secretary. By the second session he agreed to probe his feelings, which were his warning signals.

At first, victims need to concentrate on feelings of fear, hurt, and anger. In my therapy sessions, we role play ways to identify and express the feelings in a firm, straightforward way, using appropriate words and synonyms so as not to sound or feel like pouting. I explain that feelings are not meant to be lived in. They are only signals. Both my male and female clients find the role playing exercises life changing. I always suggest using these exercises in the patient's safe, present events and relationships. This brings more immediate success and, for the time being, does not bring up feelings from the past. If the trauma has just occurred, we debrief it and the resulting nightmares, first being careful not to re-traumatize the person, which may take a session or two. I ask the victim to feel the feelings, name them, and if comfortable in a few days, speak them.

Robert, like many clients, was a reluctant participant and had only come to therapy after threats of divorce by his wife. But after identifying some patterns from childhood, disclosing the nightmares, and talking about expressing feelings, he requested to return for a few more sessions. Making these connections for himself convinced him that he might learn more about ways to change those behaviors that he knew interfered with his relationships.

The danger is that without debriefing we build up the wrong kind of defenses. Covering up real feelings or exaggerating feelings may help us bluff our way through a trauma, but we fool ourselves into thinking that we have managed the trauma and its cause. We believe we have solved the problem and know what to do if it should happen again. Robert did exactly this. He thought he was the consummate problem solver. He believed that by bringing himself up he had all the answers and knew what to do in all situations, that is, until the intimacy of his marriage required more from him. His response was to withdraw and believe that he was right. He figured his only problem was his recurring nightmares. Like most of us, he had covered up his negative feelings, except for the anger which he prided himself in controlling. He made no connection between his feelings and nightmares, and what was happening in the nation and in his life.

Chapter 15

Understanding and Helping Nightmare Sufferers

*The hurt that does not find its expression in tears
may cause other organs to weep.*
—A great physician, Sir William Osler

Single vs. Multi-incident Traumas

Single-incident traumas are basically straightforward in dynamics. Although the problems of dealing with both nightmares and night terrors resulting from single-incident traumas are less complex and less difficult than those resulting from the severest of multi-incident traumas, they can vary greatly depending upon the severity of the trauma. While a child who develops nightmares due to simple fear of imagined monsters in the dark may require only simple comforting, a victim of a horrific single incident such as 9/11 will require a far more comprehensive approach.

Traumatic single incidents can be natural disasters such as earthquakes, floods, or fires. They can also include man-made events such as short-term isolated child abuse, an explosion, a severe rape or beating, or a devastating terrorist attack. Because of their short duration, single-incident traumas differ significantly from lengthy compound traumas such as the Nazi death camps, POW camps, and the type of long-term chronic child abuse that Mr. Carranza described earlier in the book. His night terrors were definitely not a product of single-incident trauma but were of the ongoing long-term variety. Many of the secondary characteristics, negative offshoots, and complications thoroughly described in chapter 6, will not develop from single-incident traumas, especially if the resulting symptoms are dealt with in a timely and effective manner. This in itself simplifies the treatment of single-incident traumas. The patient is not prone to develop overly repressed passive personality traits, deep emotional detachment, emotional blindness, an overly optimistic perspective, bronchial and sinus problems, lowered resistance to infection, memory and retention difficulties, propensity for choosing and tolerating abusive mates, or any of the other secondary problems explained earlier in the book. However, single-incident traumas may give rise to short-term aberrations and/or the magnification of existing personal struggles or interpersonal difficulties.

The victim of a single-incident trauma may begin to experience a challenge to his/her faith and trust, depression, substance abuse, fear of others and the future, impulsivity, sudden anger, moodiness, shutdown of feelings, and general anxiety. Reactions to both single and recurring incidents depend on the kinds of experiences to which a person has previously been exposed. The current atmosphere of the households and all present personal experiences also shape the individual responses of victims. Such responses, however, may also be opportunities to reexamine one's life and develop better understandings of one's values and relationships.

Single-incident-trauma-related nightmares will usually dissipate over a relatively short period of time if we have coping skills such as asking for help, reaching out to others, the ability to identify and verbalize feelings, and the willingness to talk openly about the event and our own experiences. Debriefing is the key to recovery. If we hold in our feelings and experience, we will begin to isolate and/or internalize (make personal) what has happened, which results in the negative symptoms listed above. When we share the event verbally, we correct our perceptions, determine how much it had to do with us directly, see that we are not alone in our pain, validate our own feelings along with those of others, and see that there are moments of calm and even humor. These are healing events.

Childhood reactions to a single incident may also result in trauma-related nightmares. If the cause of the nightmare is developmental rather than due to an actual event, there is no discernible reason for them. The nightmares are probably caused by the child's limited life experience, that is, his or her inability to perceive a shadow as merely a shadow. Sometimes children with emotionally safe homes may fit the personality profile of shy, sensitive, imaginative, intelligent kids and respond to mundane stimuli with nightmares or even Type A Night Terrors. As explained earlier, the sleep disruptions resulting from imagined or perceived single-incident traumas will disappear as the child's verbal acumen and growing understanding of the real world increases with age.

Debriefing

Debriefing is a process by which the sufferer is aided in exploring and examining memories of an event, so that he or she has an opportunity to move beyond denial, test the memories, and come closer to reality. Over time, this process must allow the individual to reflect on the significance of the events to his or her life and re-examine previous perceptions.

If someone presents him- or herself to you immediately after a single incident of terror or trauma, he or she needs comfort, information, and connection. In the beginning, therapy is not called for because going too deeply into feelings and re-experiencing the event will only re-traumatize the victim. What is important is listening and validating the victim's feelings. Do not negate that person's perception of the event. Help him/her find relatives, resources, directions, or professionals.

Debriefing one's feelings, thoughts, and situations at the time of a terrorizing event with personal or professional support helps immensely toward recovery. For those who are still troubled and seek help weeks or months later, it still might be best to postpone therapy and simply debrief the single incident once again.

To assess whether a faster recovery is likely, we need to take into consideration the following criteria along with the standard interview and testing information. Is there a history of trauma such as numerous family deaths over the past two years before the incident? The current trauma may cause the client to be overwhelmed, given the emotional drain from the past. Because he/she has had previous traumas, the client may also have developed good coping skills that are a foundation for healing. Does the individual have personal power such as a responsible work position, a partnership relationship, a series of successes, good language skills, insight into his/her reactions, and lack of past abuse? Determine ego strengths that provide quicker and more long-lasting recovery.

Distinguish between nightmares and Type A and B Night Terrors. Clients are not always forthcoming about abuses. Many clients report that their families are no better or worse than anyone else's. They say their parents did the best they could. They often report having a happy childhood. By asking all clients to describe their family when they were ten, to give details about their interactions and how each member dealt with anger, hurt, and fear, the therapist gets a clearer picture of their childhood and so do they. Social, emotional, and mental skills can now be assessed. Without exception, the client will discover new information that sheds light on his or her own patterns, whether healthy or not. I also ask them where in their body they feel anger, hurt, and fear. This helps me to assist them to become aware of feelings and their implicit and/or muscle memory. It gives me an opportunity to do some psycho-education about feelings and life patterns.

This approach begins the development of an understanding of the real and false self. We all create defenses as we grow up. Whatever situations we encounter, we develop skills to get through them. In the first session we begin to see what patterns we developed to survive, what facades we present, and whether they are helpful in view of what we have learned as adults. Without exception, clients can relate quickly at some level to those patterns that don't work. They just aren't sure how to re-place them.

Determining if trauma-related nightmares are a part of the client's profile can quickly point up how serious his or her reactions are to the incident. Often nightmares are one of the reasons sufferers of single incidents come in. They may not have a support system that helps them talk about the nightmares, know how to make connections between the nightmares and their experience, or know how to stop them. One way to cope with nightmares, after making connections, is to determine how victims would choose to deal with them. They may be willing to share their personal coping strategies. For example, some people find relief in aggressively confronting the objects of their fears. Just before going to bed, they will rehearse what they intend to do during the night and such preparation will cause them to sleep more restfully. This is only likely to be helpful if the incident itself has been debriefed.

Remember that these are clients without histories of chronic and/or horrendous physical, sexual, and/or emotional child abuse or chronic neglect and/or a history of living in terrorizing environments. Of course, emotionally healthy families may still have sibling problems or serious health problems, etc. Grant points out that the "quality, types and effects of various traumas must be understood so as to determine focus of treatment. Incorrect initial focus can overwhelm and/or discourage (the client)." (55, p.28)

Helping a stable, skilled person through a new horror that may challenge his/her beliefs may create a need for new ways to help his or her children, or require a new skill. But it is not the same as helping a person with previous abuse or personality disorders. Grant suggests that victims list in reverse chronological order all the traumatic experiences they have had over their lifetime. They use only titles without details and date them. (55, p.29) This is a great idea for helping the therapist and client to discuss which of these experiences are the least or most disturbing. The client can decide which one he or she would like to start with. Working on the least traumatic incident will help the therapist to assess the skills of the client for identifying feelings, using insight, making connections, identifying needs, and learning new coping methods. This effort may reveal the strength of the core personality and how the individual works with him- or herself for change and healing.

If a parent calls with the problem of a child with nightmares or night terrors, ask her to make a log of the events before the first appointment, as suggested in previous chapters. She needs to come in alone the first time for paperwork and histories, and to assess the parents' trauma background and any previous counseling. Then study the log. As therapists, many times we have asked clients to do homework only to discover later that they have not done it. Whether the log is finished and how it is finished will tell much about the involvement of the parent(s). Be sure to find out if the parents have taken the child to a physician and what that professional said or did. Many physicians say the problem will pass and there is nothing they can do.

If we determine that the family is a safe and warm environment, our greatest contribution is to share with the parents what we know about developmental and single-incident trauma-related nightmares. At the same time, the child may have responded in terror to an image or event that the parents do not see as terrorizing. A young child may not be able to verbalize what was terrorizing. The child does not know he/she is having a nightmare or a night terror attack. He/she will sit up in bed screaming. Other children may hear what is happening and tease or point out what the sufferer is doing. The parents should review the earlier chapters of this book that clarify in detail the difference between even the most horrifying of nightmares and actual night terrors.

Nightmares and night terrors are not under the control of the sufferer! This is not a behavior thought up by the child to badger the parents. Many parents who have not experienced nightmares or night terrors themselves might not understand that the sufferer does not deliberately create these events in order to get sympathy or attention. Parents need to accept and learn to cope with the fact that these intense episodes are real to the child.

Implicit nonverbal embedded defensive feelings and core constructs are formed and acted out in both trauma-related nightmares and night terrors. These feelings and constructs can be quite powerful. Researchers speak of trauma suffered by infants from birth to twenty-four months. Observing infant behavior when the caregiver leaves for ten days and the child is inadequately cared for, researchers report that infants show distinct behaviors such as refusing eye contact, turning the head, or keeping distance. Then the infant initiates connection after a few minutes. This shows defense tactics initiated by the infant for control over the caregiver. (60, p.8) This exact pattern can be observed in many unhappy adult relationships. It is a bit scary for the trained and untrained to suddenly realize that these patterns may be learned from infancy and remained unchanged. The infant implicitly learns how to control or punish the caregiver.

Soothing an infant is critical so that it can feel worthy of being comforted without resorting to defenses and other control mechanisms. Then the child can self-soothe; he/she acquires an ability to handle fear required for healthy development. Infancy and early childhood require a caregiver who sees the signs of fear. A child's first experience demands a caregiver who kneels down and talks the child through what is happening.

In *Waking the Tiger: Healing Trauma*, Peter Levine talks about working with Sammy, a two and a half year old who was traumatized by being strapped into a "pediatric papoose" so the doctor could stitch up a cut. Frightened, Sammy later began showing signs of acting out, over-controlling, and terrorizing the family. Levine helped him save Pooh Bear from under the covers as a way to help Sammy gain control over his fear of helplessness. The story is more complex, but the therapy used is dramatic in its healing powers. (61, p.256) The child is given the opportunity to build inner strength and skills that will help in later life's events. Levine offers other great ideas. He makes it clear that children often have delayed reactions. They may try to act big or to prove they are strong. Instead they, like adults, need debriefing, or a chance later to express their feelings and talk about what happened. Levine describes this process well.

Whether a child has nightmares due to actual single incidents or to misperceptions of mundane events, the therapy is the same. The child needs routine, particularly at bedtime, enough sleep, support for feelings, and ways to gain confidence in facing fear. Fear not dealt with becomes generalized anxiety over time, and the mind struggles to explain the anxiety the body is experiencing. Any new fear adds to the anxiety. No skill is developed to stop the cycle.

Processing Trauma

If debriefing does not occur or is not successful, the overwhelming sensory input becomes a part of long-term memory. Trauma-related nightmares, along with unhealthy patterns of all kinds, are a great tool for uncovering these memories. It is imperative that we first understand how these memories are formed and how early this can happen. In addition, knowing that feelings are instrumental in what parts of memory are stored, we must be clear about the significance of feelings in everyday life as well as in memory storage.

The processing of any event begins with a specific memory through an individual's senses, perceptions, previous experiences, beliefs, intuitions, and both implicit and explicit memories. If we have been through traumas before, we may have developed skills to handle them. On the other hand, if the previous traumas had not provided us with ways to function in such events, we might handle the current trauma poorly. I have found that many clients have a problem with bereavement. If the person was brought up with rituals and family support, grieving becomes a natural process of loss. However, if the client has been told that crying is not acceptable and loss is something one gets over automatically in due time, the unresolved grieving has consequences years later, showing itself in the avoidance of signs of illness or negative feelings and the inability to have close relationships.

Trauma brings up many personal issues. Suddenly significant others and/or the world are no longer safe. This may shift the way we perceive ourselves. Did we cause or contribute to the events? Are we responsible for the losses we bear? The answers to such questions may lead us to perceive ourselves as bad, wrong, guilty, inferior, or shameful, creating the belief that we're not good enough and significantly lowering our self-esteem. Our world-view and self-view become limited and focused on potential threats to our safety and comfort. Gone is the freedom to risk, explore, experiment, or expand emotional or social skills. The stage is set for trauma-related nightmares that result from faulty and fragmented memories.

A traumatic event is stored in long-term memory by the emotional strength the event creates—an image alive with nonverbal warnings. Imagine how many people remember years later what embarrassed them in childhood. They can still experience the feelings created by this seemingly insignificant occurrence. How much more embedded would be memories of sexual, physical, or emotional abuse! The nervous system is chemically changed and holds such images until dealt with. These memories can be triggered by a myriad of reminders, from a smell, to a touch, a person, a voice, a setting, or a movie. Traumatized persons may not even know they have experienced a trigger, but the images or feelings arise in nightmares and daydreams, or impinge on current thoughts. The most severe of these traumas may be suppressed and not remembered consciously. It is such suppressed traumatic events that can lead to actual night terrors. Re-experiencing the event may be the mind and body's way of reminding us that there are dangers. Such sleep thinking images sabotage our beliefs, emotions, and behaviors.

When severely traumatized by brutal events, the body responds to protect itself, just as it does in stress or embarrassment. The parasympathetic nervous system causes the body to be ready for fight or flight, basically a shock reaction. Debriefing a nightmare can unlock the shock and fear. Using feelings to hold down reactions burns energy. This is why stress exhausts us. An example is when a spouse cannot let go of an image after demanding that the other spouse tell all the details of his/her partner's affair. My client, Betty, agreed to work with her husband to put their marriage on a better path, yet she kept badgering him about his affair because images kept creeping into her thoughts and dreams. Clearly the images helped her to revisit her anger and thus protect her from "giving in" or trusting him and getting hurt again. She complained about being emotionally exhausted.

By processing the daydreaming or nightmare images, putting them in a context of new information and beliefs, the individual can begin to heal. By bringing the images and feelings to awareness or consciousness, Betty could control her responses. How did Betty see her relationship now that they were trying to communicate more? How might the couple reawaken their passion for each other? If they were to dream together, what would they dream? How would they make it come true? The memories must come to awareness or they cannot be resolved, reconciled, or restructured.

Remember, night terrors occur during the deepest slow wave non-REM (NREM) sleep. A victim of night terrors may have minimal or no recall of content. On the other hand, dreams and nightmares occur during REM sleep when the person can remember or be trained to remember the content and some sense can be made of the images or the sensations. Sometimes the sensations are so powerful during REM sleep that the dreams or nightmares are interrupted. This is thought by some to impede the process the brain is using to "file" or "heal" trauma. Therapists need to consider this differentiation to better determine any treatment plan.

Trauma-related nightmares give us good examples of how underlying, unconscious responses can disrupt our lives without our conscious control. With the use of spectrometer scans, neurobiologists have a clearer picture literally and figuratively of the effect of trauma on the brain. The neurons and the release of chemicals are physically altered by stress, trauma, and terror. Parnell wrote, "Trauma, particularly during the early stages of brain development, impairs mental and emotional functioning and affects physiology far more than we realized and for a much longer time. Trauma memory is stored differently than ordinary memory. [The latter], stored in the right hemisphere in fragmented, unintegrated form, [is] separate from the brain's language center." (62, p. 8) She continued by describing implicit and explicit memory and pointing out that, in early childhood, schemas of the self and world are developed through the sensory-motor systems. All is based on needs and whether those needs are met. This is an unconscious process embedded in the emotional apparatus of the brain.

Explicit memory is narrative memory that can be explained through words and stories. There is a sense of self, a knowing. These are memories that go from short- to long-term and the individual is aware of the process.

From birth to three the child has "infantile amnesia," because parts of the brain have yet to mature and most memory is implicit. Such memories of trauma are not communicated through words or stories. They are unconsciously expressed and acted out by the body in symptoms such as tight muscles, nervous stomach, and headaches. Research on infancy begins to highlight how this occurs and how significant this implicit memory process is to our entire life. We can see this in research on infants functioning on implicit memory and their relationship to a caregiver. Could implicit, somatic memory provide images and feelings for some nightmares, and explicit memory provide the story content for others?

Nightmares, especially relating to feelings such as fear and anxiety, can relate back to infancy. Realizing how early memory is activated deepens our understanding of the significance of the connection between feelings and memories.

Jacovitz and Hazen in *Attachment Disorganization* wrote of

the central role of fear in attachment between infants and care-givers. These attachments form the foundation of a healthy emotional and physical life. The purpose of this infant-caregiver relationship is to provide a safe environment. The mutual relational dance—functional or dysfunctional—develops habitual patterns that will allow the participants to survive in their relationship. These patterns serve to defend us when, later on, danger presents itself and triggers fear. Research on attachment lists as fear-provoking: separation from the caregiver, hunger, being in strange surroundings, fatigue, and whatever distresses the infant.

When the caregiver is sensitive and responsive by meeting the needs of the child rather than the needs of the parent, the infant feels secure and learns it can rely on safety provided by the care-giver, gain trust in the environment, and develop a positive inner structure. This allows the infant to attach, to develop confidence in the self, and to maintain overall functioning. Who we are begins in infancy, not at three, five, or seven! We can no longer afford to write off infancy and early childhood. (60, pp.4–6) "Because these processes function largely outside consciousness (implicit memory, muscle memory), internal working models tend to be resistant to change." (60, p.6) We need to know this process in the infant brain because it is easier to be proactive than reactive. In other words, preventing bad habits and patterns is easier than fixing them. Changing established unconscious troublesome patterns such as stuffing feelings or raging takes hard work. Because such patterns are developed over long periods of time, any recognition of patterns becomes a challenge to the core of the person. Harmful patterns can be avoided by a caregiver who fulfills a child's emotional and physical needs.

When there is chronic distress in the lives of infants, they tend to behave with push-pull behaviors—"angry resistance . . . with contact-maintaining behaviors." (60, p.10) An infant may reach out by hanging on, then letting go and hanging over the care-giver's arm, by maintaining eye contact, then breaking it, or by cooing, then fussing. This has unnerved more than one parent!

What kinds of parental behaviors bring about these patterns

that can last long into adulthood? The parent may not have resolved his/her own childhood trauma and fears of intimacy. The caregiver may have suffered the death of a loved one, may be in mourning and have "unresolved loss when he or she displays lapses in the monitoring or reasoning, discourse, or behavior." (60, p.87) The caregiver may act out his/her own aggression. Some behaviors may not be seen as abusive, but in repetitive, chronic relationships they can cause defensive reactions that become patterns. I can just hear the responses of many clients. "That's the way I was treated and I turned out fine." Without exception I could see many ways these persons are having serious interpersonal relationship problems. Such learned patterns, beliefs, defenses, and perceptions are stored chemically in the brain and give us a sense of who we are and how we behave in response to internal and external events.

Nature and nurture are not either/or processes. Who we are is tucked away in the different kinds of memory that have been programmed through the years along with our hardwiring or genetic uniqueness. Yet both can be modified or changed. Like our bodies and our environment, we are constantly changing. Though they know better, many clients want their lives to function successfully using the defenses and knowledge they already have. It is not easy to learn and grow if one is closed and defensive. Yet, when clients get new information, it helps them make some changes they can see as helpful. Working with trauma-related nightmares facilitates this process. I have found clients particularly intrigued with their dreams and nightmares.

Memory is tricky business. Explicit memory relies on one's awareness and perceptions. These determine what is allowed into the system, to what degree it is fragmented, how it is interpreted, and how it is recalled or repressed. Our emotional and sensory input ends up in implicit or muscle memory. All of this is affected by and impacts both body and mind. It seems to help clients to learn that we store feelings in part of the brain and that these stored feelings can be triggered, making situations more volatile. The same is true with sharing information about stress chemicals.

Some readers may have read Sapolsky's book, *Why Zebras*

Don't Have Ulcers. If you have, you know its significance in explaining the inevitable interaction between stress, the body, the mind, and our behavior. If you have not, it is highly recommended reading.

The stress hormones, glucocorticoids, can give new meaning to the reality that too much of a good thing can be bad. Not attended to, or over time, glucorcorticoids may damage neurons and interrupt the release and take-up of neurotransmitters in the brain, which create nonfunctional behaviors and thought patterns. Such changes include depression, anhedonia (inability to feel pleasure), learned helplessness, psychomotor retardation (inability to get out of bed), alterations in appetite, disrupted sleep patterns, and an inability of the hormone system to return to balance, all of which contributes to disease.

Over years of studying glucocorticoid levels in wild monkey troupes, Sapolsky found that balanced hormones such as norepinephrine, seratonin, and dopamine provide normal responses to stress. This allows the monkeys to (1) tell the difference between threatening and neutral interactions, (2) take the initiative if the situation is obviously threatening, (3) tell whether they have won or lost, and (4) find ways to release any frustration. When we as humans respond appropriately to a given situation because we use our emotional energy to assess and respond, our physical and psychological abilities are working for us.

When the monkeys' stress hormones were out of balance over time, as in people who are intense workaholics or those with generalized anxiety, these animals (1) were unable to keep competition in perspective, (2) withdrew from social interaction, and (3) became unaware of life improving or worsening. These results parallel what happens when a human can no longer "think straight" or when he or she perceives life through a filter of depression or anger. Though it is hard to believe that anyone could discover these truths in monkeys, reading Sapolsky's book will provide proof of how the body and the mind work together in the African or the cement jungle.

To believe that symptoms such as nightmares resulting from a trauma or a horrendous childhood come from a particular genetic predisposition is to misunderstand the use of the word "inherited." The confusion is critical because, if one believes the symptoms of traumatic events or chronic abuse to be genetic, one may believe one's self helpless to overcome these patterns.

Many believe that feelings of anxiety are normal in their family and that they are genetic, therefore, unchangeable. Inherited predisposition may be seen in several ways. If we consider stress as a symptom, we might be living with it because of the lack of skills to cope with situations at home or work. Stress may even come from past generations of alcohol abuse. The resulting behaviors, say, of anger, have been passed on as patterns of rage and stress. We certainly can genetically inherit family characteristics such as a more high-wired nervous system or a slow metabolic system. We can get nongenetic chemical imbalances at birth that may result in stress. For example, the pregnant woman who drinks or takes drugs can predispose her fetus to many future maladies or defects. Living in stress-filled neighborhoods or stress-filled homes can keep our stress hormones out of balance and cause permanent genetic and physical alterations. But, like the differences in our biological makeup or our particular home or neighborhood, we must cope with what we have been dealt. Knowing how we develop memories, how we become who we are, what our patterns are, and that we can change them for a better life, we are empowered in our own journey.

The Effects of Culture

Not all victims subjected to horror and terror are so traumatized that it interferes with their lives. Yet, to determine who is most likely to be significantly wounded by horrific events, we need to look at the victim's family, gender, and culture, as well as other circumstances that go beyond the individual. Earlier I have specifically covered caregivers and the family in general. But I need to be clear that understanding how an individual, or even a country, responds to abuse or terror is complex. It seems to be a human trait that we think others should believe and act like us. As a therapist I know only too well that working with psychologically wounded people from different cultures can be difficult unless I know something about that culture. I must be sensitive to what I don't know and then empower the client to educate me.

Asking about dreams, nightmares, or night terrors might feel intrusive in some cultures and very respected in others. I get around some of this by asking clients specifically to tell me if they are feeling uncomfortable about any of my questions. I also ask them if they are comfortable working with someone outside of their culture. Though I have never had anyone become offended, I stay as sensitive as possible to the client's reticence to questions. I always keep in mind that this reluctance could have a basis in the client's cultural heritage.

In such a diverse culture as the United States, we must realize that stress can be caused by the conflicts that differences create. There are family as well as country, religious, and ethnic culture issues. The family culture results from the beliefs, ethnicity, behaviors, and experiences of previous generations. Husband and wife reflect the heritage from which they come. These heritages often conflict during marriages, particularly in parenting. With trauma-related nightmare victims, I am particularly aware of patterns passed on to unknowing, unsuspecting infants and that are projected as truth when the children are growing. The majority of my time as a therapist is spent in helping clients to see that there are alternatives to the ways they have learned. The difficulties for the client lie in the clash or acceptance arising from the overall world culture versus regional and ethnic differences.

Terrance Real in *I Don't Want to Talk About It* pointed out, "As a culture historically dominated by male values, we have always tended, and still tend, to deny vulnerability, and consequently, to deny the existence of trauma." No doubt this cultural view had been strengthened in America by having no enemy on our homeland in living memory even through two world wars. When an enemy managed to penetrate our boundaries on September 11, we were totally unprepared intellectually and emotionally.

In addition, there exist numerous sociology books naming other critical cultural changes affecting the ways we cope or don't cope with trauma. The 1950s are long past, yet we seem to hold on to fifties values while trying to fit into the new technoculture. In *Why We Don't Talk to Each Other Anymore: The De-Voicing of Society*, John Locke explored factors that are driving us apart. He proposed that it takes some type of disaster or other crisis to even get us to talk to our neighbors. Culturally we have developed an environment replete with technology touted as saving us time, energy, and efficiency. In practice, much of technology has been interpreted not as a tool to enhance who we are but rather as a substitute for personal interaction, particularly at the emotional connecting level. I have seen an increase in individual and couple problems due to cyberspace. More and more, people are having relationships with the computer or with others through e-mail, having cybersex with strangers, relating to pornography on the computer, reading headlines or watching news that delivers information in thirty seconds to five minutes, and being targeted for products as an anonymous part of a particular group. I have also seen more and more people being relocated by job necessity and/or living alone in bigger and better homes. Locke quoted Evan Schwartz, an author for *Wired Magazine,* as writing that America will be "the first society with Attention Deficit Disorder . . . the official brain syndrome for the information age."

Locke, unlike sociologists writing about the dumbing down of America, was concerned about connection. We learn by being face-to-face. We pick up emotional nuances that cannot be expressed in writing. I relate to his view when I see the increase in extreme behaviors. We seem simply to have little time for nuances. People feel there is no time for relating, much less for figuring out what the other person is saying. Spontaneous individual perception, whether right or wrong, and external anger or its counterpart, depression, become the filter for relationships—a far cry from connecting. All forms of media discourage taking time for such considerations.

When Locke discussed television, I fondly remembered asking a family if they talked to each other. They were adamant about their ability to communicate. I asked them to describe the times when they talked. With pride they agreed it was during the commercials, while they were eating dinner. I let what they said hang in the air for a pregnant minute and then asked if they solved problems during that time. They stared at each other, then looked at me, and then we all laughed. Sudden insight is a great thing!

We are socially oriented and need relationships. In a society that is not safe—one that is argumentative, critical, anti-vulnerability, materialistic, and dehumanizing—we can only imagine how abused and traumatized people feel. As long as there is a common enemy, as there was on September 11, we can turn these societal characteristics to our benefit. However, such behaviors are disastrous in families and in the community. This brings us back to Real's statement that our history has determined our gender roles. "The forces of gender are far more complex than a simple male-female dichotomy suggests." (63, p.167) However, we cannot deny that much of what we consider the male role and masculinity predetermines our beliefs about both men and women.

Robert was certainly caught in the culture not only of the nation but also of the corporation. The skills he learned among male teams in high school and college and the male corporate hierarchy provided him with great success in business but not at home. The home culture has a different set of expectations, ones which are often influenced by the woman's traditional role as homemaker.

Healthy Responses to Trauma

A key to all healthy coping with normal or horrendous events is how and if we value feelings. Emotionally healthy people use their feelings as thermometers for what is happening in the atmosphere at home and work, as well as in any event and/or relationship. Feelings keep us in the moment. If we let the moment go by, we may get off the track by hearing something other than the real meaning or the immediate concern. We can be quick to jump to wrong conclusions if we bypass the moment of feeling.

We can help parents understand the role of feelings in their relationships which help them be sensitive to and validate the feelings of their children. In view of all of this information, I am not saying that we must spend a great deal of time dealing with the client's history. On the other hand, his or her history remains a hotbed of connections, patterns, beliefs, and potential insights. In an interview for *Marriage & Family: A Christian Journal*, Dr. Susan M. Johnson said, "I might use the past to validate how someone is in the present." (64, p.117) As co-creator with Leslie Greenberg of emotionally focused therapy (EFT), Dr. Johnson's purpose was to get couples to connect through staying with emotions as central to relationships. Feelings are the body mechanisms that tell us an immediate event is important to us and that we'd better pay attention to it. Dr. Johnson saw insight as tangential to the business of resolving couples' differences. She asserted that all persons want others to know them as they are, to know how they see things and accept their need to feel safe in a relationship, as well as to recognize that these things are not negotiable.

When feelings are buried, they become implicit memory. These "feeling memories" can be easily triggered by other traumas. This process happens to us all, but if we are to maintain a balanced life, we must respect and acknowledge our feelings as well as learn to verbalize them at the time they occur. Again, sharing all kinds of feelings is the foundation of intimacy and protection against self-abuse and abuse by others. Feelings are to the human being as signal lights are to a complex and overcrowded intersection. Pay no attention and you may very well die emotionally and certainly relationally. Therefore, as I am emphasizing throughout, a healthy response to trauma and its resulting symptoms must include a major focus on unearthing and dealing with our true feelings.

Chapter 16

The Healing Process

I found in the midst of winter there is in me an
invincible spring.
—Albert Camus

The Importance of Grieving

Sudden severe traumas and disasters are especially devastating because they represent such a great threat to our own sense of control and security. September 11, 2001, was a unique example of this in that, unlike other catastrophes, it challenged a nation's belief in itself, its collective comfort, and its conception of battle. We all felt invaded and violated. We were numb, disbelieving, disoriented, and looking around as though we might catch a glimpse of our reality—life, as we knew it.

The shock of it all tumbles into feelings of fear, helplessness, and denial. Then someone speaks to us, runs past us, screams for help, or just says, "Can you believe it?" Pulled back to our senses, we move to action. We call loved ones, we do our job, we lend a hand, we sit on the curb to recover, we say, "This is terrible, what can I do?" In a dreamlike state we begin to realize the enormity of it all and feel overwhelmed. But for the next three or four days there is so much to do—keep up with routine, give assistance to others, make necessary arrangements, keep abreast of what is happening, make plans, and contact resources. Then it hits! The grieving process has begun.

Every culture has struggled over the centuries with loss of life, loss of ideals, natural disasters, battles, and sudden change. But, why must we actually experience grief? Why not suppress it or "just get on with our lives"? Even though grief is a negative and painful emotion, it is necessary because it is the essential process of overcoming and successfully adjusting to loss. Grief helps us to make connections, find meaning, and open ourselves to deep feelings and higher values.

Common sense leads us to avoid pain. But pain is an integral part of coping with the real world and dealing with what life brings—the ups and downs of daily living. It is this process of grieving that prepares us to heal from disasters and catastrophes, both national and personal. How well each of us will respond to an event and how well we will traverse grief are determined by our own life experiences and coping skills. Physically, mentally, emotionally, and spiritually, we are built to survive, thrive, attach, and hope. To avoid grieving is to avoid life.

The avoidance of the grieving process invites trauma-related nightmares and other symptoms by which the sleeping brain insists that we address and resolve the tragedy. Memories of tragedies like 9/11 carry powerful feelings that subtly haunt our conscious and unconscious. It takes time and direction to turn grieving into healing. Failing to tackle our own mental and emotional responses results in acting-out behaviors, whether asleep or awake.

Earlier in the book Mr. Carranza talked about the Chowchilla kidnapping, which is a prime example of a single-incident trauma. Four years after that event, Nader reported that the children had repetitive nightmares, 57 percent had night terrors, 30 percent had modified kidnapping dreams and 52 percent had disguised dreams (other theme nightmares). She also cited another incident where a child acted out her repressed feelings after being injured and traumatized during a tornado. The child became aggressive toward her mother and had nightmares. After a hurricane an adolescent had hurricane nightmares for two months in which time his mother didn't allow him to talk about it. (56, pp.14, 15) Trauma-related nightmares are a personalization of the event.

Researchers are already documenting nightmares and other responses of children and adults as they recover from September 11.

In order for effective healing to take place, steps must be taken toward the reestablishment of health. First, each of us needs to reexamine our feelings and perceptions of what happened. Second, we must determine what the experience has told us about our own lives, strengths, and weaknesses. Third, as a nation as well as individuals, we must decide, according to what we experienced, who we want to be and how we want to act. Fourth, individually and as a nation, we need to assess our resources for any eventuality. And fifth, we need to develop increased resilience and inner faith so that we can find ways to move ahead regardless of what happens in the future.

Children and adults have their own individual healing time. Both children and adults need solace, comfort, and validation for the first three or four weeks. Without validation, fear is denied. It explodes as anger. Those who have been through trauma before may be more volatile and angry because the previous events were not handled well. Others who are trained or have learned from past traumas may seem unusually calm and deliberate. This does not mean that they lack fear or compassion.

"Dreams may both replicate aspects of the traumatic experience and incorporate psychodynamic issues, for example, issues of protection, betrayal, loss or accountability." (56, p.19) This is true for children, adults, and nations. After 9/11 our nation experienced these same issues: loss of protection, a sense of betrayal by government agencies, loss of control, comfort, and complacency, and a need to determine who was and will be accountable for keeping us safe. This points again to the complexity of healing from trauma. It is not merely overcoming fear. Beliefs, faith, possibilities, and goals are challenged.

Denial is often the first sign that grieving is occurring. When our beliefs are challenged our inclination is to hang on to them more tightly. But 9/11 pointed out the futility of clinging to beliefs that were unexamined and, we thought, unchanging. We all now feel a scary vulnerability. Our ideals and assumptions about ourselves have been shattered. We are not omnipotent; our soil is not sacrosanct. Yet accepting this new reality is a big part of our hope for healing. Each person takes in and perceives the trauma in his/her own way. Healing requires sharing and accepting many perceptions to realize the most objective reality. This provides a concept or structure into which we can stabilize our experience with that of others. It is the beginning of seeing the "bigger picture." From this we can assess the real damage and determine what we need to do next.

Another common reaction in grieving is anger. The idea of exacting revenge on the perpetrators may come up in trauma-related nightmares. Such sleep disturbances point to issues needing resolution. Often our anger is misdirected because we are not sure at whom to be angry. After 9/11, some were angry at select foreign nations, certain ethnic immigrants, or our own intelligence organizations and politicians.

Another feeling in the grieving process along with denial and anger is guilt or condemning oneself for being involved in the event. "If only I had left on time I would have been safe." "I should have arrived earlier to save my friend." Guilt may show up in nightmares. Some people may dream of preventing the event or rescuing others. The purpose of both anger and guilt is to help us determine what the trauma meant to us.

Another evidence of grieving is depression. Denial, anger, and guilt often turn into depression. If these feelings are suppressed, they can be acted out in several ways, all of which are signals of unresolved thoughts and perceptions. The resultant behaviors may be aggression, violence, withdrawal, or passivity, depending on the individual's personality. If feelings of shame, guilt, jealousy, anger, or violence from the past have been suppressed, such feelings may be re-triggered or magnified by a new trauma and may appear in nightmares. Stress in other parts of the person's life may also result in sleep disruption.

The feeling of depression is normal and natural if used as a signal to pay attention to identifying a problem. Depression slows down the body, mind, and emotions. This makes us withdraw enough from our routine to cope with loss. Some animals howl and sway over their dead much like people at a funeral or wake. But people, being complex, need to take time to "sit with their pain," cry, be alone, and accept the reality. This is most important when dealing with extreme national or personal tragedies. Most will begin bereavement with shock that normally takes three days to a week to overcome. Some may start with denial or anger. In grieving, some may go into depression first, particularly if they have been overwhelmed with other traumas.

All of this emotion may appear in trauma-related nightmares, and the content may change as these emotions change. By remembering the content, identifying the feelings experienced in the nightmare or flashback, and making connections to what has and is happening in one's life, it is possible to determine what is most upsetting and what needs to be more closely examined for its significance to one's personal adjustment and relationships. As terrible as it is, incorporating the insights and meanings of the trauma into our beliefs and necessary skills brings us to full healing.

To some degree, we are all walking wounded. Our personalities are full of scars; many of them date from very early childhood or even infancy. We should not despair. Our traumas may be our most effective tools in the process of reeducating ourselves to handle life better. Probably the most difficult task in healing remains the realization that trauma is one of our best teachers. Conversely, mixing denial with a failure to learn from traumatic experiences is following a proven recipe for a lifetime of tragedy.

Resilience

Not everyone who experiences trauma, tragedy, or disaster will have trauma-related nightmares. And in general, nightmares seem to lessen as we get older. Perhaps this is one reason, when adults do have them, the symptoms may be particularly poignant. Nightmares can help to make connections to old memories and sensations that lie deep in the shadows of our personality. But if these connections, which were not made at the time the trauma occurred, go unresolved, they become the hidden elements of sleep thinking that can cause a greater sensitivity to later life traumas, making one prone to develop recurring nightmares. As with 9/11 or any traumatic event, if it occurs after previous major life trauma(s), then the negative sleep repercussions will be more severe and obvious. Firemen and rescue workers with less severe sleep symptoms may be persons who have experienced only minor previous psychological wounds. Those with more dramatic sleep symptoms may be persons who were already hypersensitive because of severe earlier life traumas. As explained before, severely abused children can develop night terrors in childhood and throughout adolescence. Then, upon moving away from their abusive homes in early adulthood, there is a lull in their night terror activity. Later, after marrying a highly abusive spouse, the problem may explode with more ferocity and frequency than ever before. This is a prime example of the latent compounded effects of extreme trauma.

Those who do not have recurrent, repetitive, or flashback nightmares after experiencing intense trauma may also be those who have developed skills over a lifetime that allow them to handle the worst life scenarios. Developing skills does not mean shutting out feelings or experiences. On the contrary, these are more likely to be people who are open, set boundaries, look for meanings, make connections to what they have been through before, put the experience into perspective regarding the future, and choose how they will handle the new life created by the terror they have survived. In such cases we are most likely to be talking about older persons whose lives have required them to make adjustments through a number of tragedies.

The resilient adult has the ability to respond to and incorporate trauma into his or her reality. Put simply, it is a better than average ability to overcome tragedy. Such people have learned to cope with trouble as soon as possible. During their lives they have discovered that trauma not healed can cause attention, anxiety, and conduct disorders, as well as marital, learning, and substance abuse problems. Resilient adults have been described in research as having, among other attributes, a positive sense of self, an ability to absorb information and take suggestions, and the capacity to create positive visions and meanings from both positive and negative life experiences. They also possess the abilities to embrace change, become educated, sustain positive relationships and support systems, and to continually work for a more positive interpersonal world. (65, p.20) Further, these adults are genuine, optimistic, and friendly; they expect their efforts to have positive outcomes, are clear about their feelings, take responsibility for their mistakes and correct them, and face conflict. Higgins goes on to write that these people are not saints. They can be ill tempered, argumentative, inconsiderate, and even rude at times. They have self-worth issues and must struggle to uphold their integrity, but they "maintain high self-esteem regarding their own executive and interpersonal competence, believe that they deserve to be loved and feel that their trials made them far more than they might have been otherwise." (65, p.21)

All of these characteristics require an internal locus of control. Viscott wrote, "Peace of mind comes with self-acceptance . . . the gift you give yourself." (59, p.352) The individual must manage him- or herself rather than feel entitled to the generosity of others. An external locus utilizes judging, blaming, and manipulating others to make one's own life better. Robert was a good example of one who had external locus, as was Lucy (discussed in earlier chapters). When 9/11 occurred, Robert was having marital problems and was horrified by what he thought was his wife's whimpering about being taken over by terrorists. She was furious at his response because he showed no consideration for her feelings. A partner with internal locus would support the other's view, then add his/her own view without passing judgment.

Much of the problem in healing trauma arises from the self-protective memory fragments of the event(s). We see the traumatic event(s) from our position at the time and no one else can exactly stand in our shoes. To help cope with terror, we allow into our consciousness only what makes sense to us. We begin to construct our own story, even incorporating what we read in newspapers or see on television. At best this results in a partial reality of the actual terror. Such perceptions are driven by high emotion. The telling of the "story" to desensitize the recollections is the goal, not determining whether the elements are "real."

When we perceive memory as a "mixed bag" of information, images, and responses, we open the door to freedom. "The key to transforming trauma is to move slowly in the direction of flexibility and spontaneity." (61, p.215) Healing requires being open to new interpretations, learning, and insights. Otherwise, we live in a past that has become our present reality. Moving on takes time and work, but trying to be safe by standing still wastes energy. Action creates energy.

Robert needed to give himself permission to heal rather than continually repeat his ways of thinking and behaving, which failed in both home and work relationships. He obsessed about financial success in closing deals with strangers. He protected himself from his failures by perceiving others as failing him. After all, how could they not see it his way when authorities and customers praised his "people skills." His fragmented memories were emotionally selected to avoid the pain of realizing his lack of skills with any long-term relationships. So he worked harder and longer with strangers and made more money to reinforce his belief that those close to him needed to change. His reaction to his wife about 9/11 was but one symptom of his selective views. He freely commiserated with those who got angry, a feeling with which he was comfortable.

Robert didn't feel he had options and choices. His way was the only way, even though it wasn't working. Conversely, resilient persons are convinced they can choose, that they can create their own lives. Survivors learn from coping successfully with trauma that there can be a more humane life. They have been to hell and ultimately learn that there can be a better future. But one has to work for improvement and not just wish that others would make it happen for them.

One way to prove that all this is possible is to manage one's trauma-related nightmares. Higgins reported on a person who brought a comforting image into her nightmares. (65, p.181) She practiced that image until it was able to comfort and soothe her fears during her nightmares. Dr. Barry Krakow on ABC's *20/20* program called this process "imagery rehearsal therapy" and said it had a 90 percent success rate, even among persons who had nightmares about 9/11. This of course doesn't change underlying causes, but it does give relief to those who don't have other symptoms. Realizing that we can change our daily and nightly reactions will help the resilient to move forward.

Healthy survivors are converted to the process of improving, learning, and balancing their lives day by day. They can accept their sadness over losing idealistic dreams and take responsibility for moving forward. They can risk compassion. Healthy survivors also see the dark side, but, knowing they have choices, they are less likely to live in denial or have fragmented memories.

Abusers believe they are the only ones who hurt. Without compassion, they continue to hurt others as they demonstrate varying degrees of psychopathology. Keeping anger inside results in long-suffering guilt and shame. Being hurt doesn't justify hurting others. The unhealthy will continue to vilify the healthy and deny all responsibility for their behavior. In contrast, thrivers live their integrity in the face of hurt from others. Appropriate anger is the energy that helps set boundaries. The healthy set limits so as not to allow harmful behavior, thereby creating a safer environment in which to thrive rather than merely survive. The thriver does not proselytize or become obsessed with "saving" the abuser. He or she does not condone evil but rather recognizes it, and stands firm in his or her convictions. He/she is able to keep moving forward even while knowing and honoring deep sadness. Healthy survivors know that neither families, nations, churches, nor banks are automatically "safe." Safety is internal. The thriver is able to forgive when recognition, remorse, and reparation are forthcoming. (65, p.296) Higgins sums it up by indicating that the healthy survivor does not unconsciously collaborate with abusers by "thinking that the work of recovery can be avoided by extending unearned forgiveness to them; and putting inordinate amounts of energy into forgiving abuse or abandonment when it could be invested in self-growth." (65, p.299)

Abusers, as well as terrorists, usually are either unwilling to admit to their abuse or are arrogant in their justification of violent, harmful behavior. Earned forgiveness requires the abuser to admit openly his or her actions and then drastically and clearly change his or her behaviors over an extended period of time. Such change is virtually impossible with the conscienceless, unrepentant psychopath. In most cases, they will persistently continue to abuse. The resilient survivor will recognize this, accept it, and then move on with life.

Preparing for Treatment

For all clients, but especially for the traumatized, the first job of the therapist is to provide a safe environment. Victims have lost their sense of safety, trust, and confidence, as well as some of their cherished beliefs. They are hyperalert to anything they think might threaten them, however small. Some will not seek help for months or years after a terrorizing or other severely traumatic event. It is imperative to remember that when being asked to help a trauma-related nightmare sufferer, this hypersensitivity will signal any disingenuousness on the part of the therapist. My traumatized clients often questioned me if I so much as looked away or raised an eyebrow. One client told me well into the second stage of therapy that the most important responses I gave were communicated by my body language.

The therapist must be ready to be real, vulnerable, honest, and professional. Both client and therapist must join in the therapeutic alliance. I see this as a mandate to set aside my expectations and even my techniques until I get a solid understanding of the needs of the client. This, to me, means being theoretically eclectic, holding in abeyance my schemas and techniques until the client is able to articulate his or her needs and goals. I respond with what will best help the individual based on his or her goals and cooperation in achieving them. There is no mystery in my interactions because I believe the client is going to have to live his/her life outside of my office. True change is a process of making and carrying out choices, the success of which relies on willingness to risk in some degree and on having a sense of self-advocacy. This may mean taking very short strides or longer strides, depending upon the client's ego strength. But then, that's how mountains are eventually climbed.

In working with trauma victims of any kind it is important to identify how the client's past and present environment affects his/her responses to the event. Environmental factors may include abandonment, an abusive upbringing, being raised in a high crime, fear-filled neighborhood, national events, terrorist acts, and personal fears and/or tragedies. The victim may have experienced racial or life-style prejudices, been affected by gender expectations, or been a member of a particular culture or religion. A professional will make disastrous mistakes if these influences have not been deciphered and considered as the backdrop for the client's reactions to trauma.

Robert's Therapy

In beginning Robert's therapy, we needed to take into account not only all the factors discussed in the preceding section but also that he had led an exceptionally disturbed life. The horror of 9/11 added to his many existing problems. He had never been able to cope with his past, exhibited extreme anxiety and anger, and suffered from PTSD. Since the present account centers around a man, it should be pointed out that the primary difference in working with a female client would be the need to recognize that usually a woman's equivalent to a man's anger is being "emotional." We can't live in feelings; we use them to help identify what is happening—good or bad. Both women and men need to learn to manage rather than manipulate relationships through feelings. Consequently, everybody needs to solve relational problems daily.

Because of Robert's work success, he had many reasons to avoid therapy. This he had done throughout the years of his marriage. However, in his own way he loved his wife and children enough to prevent an imminent divorce. His wife had been passive until she gave him three months to begin learning to be her partner, not her boss, and to be sensitive, not angry. This and an increase in his nightmares because of 9/11 prompted him to seek therapy.

Following are the stages of his therapy. They demonstrate one of the ways a professional might work with someone who had serious symptoms before the trauma or didn't respond to support afterward. I have already described the initial session in previous chapters.

Immediate therapeutic goals for Robert would be to prevent escalation of emotions, build on his skills, and develop ways to decrease the nightmares. Long-term goals would center around helping him gain inner strength and control over himself, gain skills related to self-expression of negative feelings, acquire a more realistic rather than perfectionistic view of himself and others, develop new insights from the trauma, alter his present view of his past, and apply his new discoveries to real scenarios. Throughout the therapy process, clients must be asked how the last week went, what worked, what didn't, and what insights were acquired. We all learn from day-to-day experiences but we seldom ask ourselves these questions.

Each session must provide continuing management of symptoms. For Robert, this meant practicing and reporting ways of soothing himself to lower his stress responses that in turn lessened his symptoms. He also paid attention to the feelings and messages in his nightmares. This, along with attempts at altering them, succeeded with only a few relapses. The relapses allowed us to find new and creative ways to respond to stress and anxiety.

This began his journey toward relieving long-buried pain and gaining real inner confidence rather than exaggerated outer confidence.

Each mid-stage session began with trauma debriefing, which had started after the initial session. The emphasis now was on feelings, meanings, and learning rather than the actual experiences of 9/ll and his failing marriage. We could begin to explore healthful patterns from his past while looking at both old and new ones. Robert could now relate stories from his early childhood that held connections for him. His parents were very critical and gave him a constant fear of being out of control and a sense of not being good enough. He remembered feeling the same kinds of anxiety and helplessness because of 9/11. The criticisms were so severe that he wasn't sure he had the right to be a person. As the sessions progressed, he began to realize his whole identity was in the positive reactions provided by strangers and authorities.

Throughout these sessions, I helped Robert to identify his feelings, to use his salesman skills for romance, to discover ways to counter the self-criticism in his own mind, to be genuine, to relieve his anxiety, and to allow himself to be as successful as he wished. Toward the end of his sessions, Robert admitted he didn't want to be a workaholic and that he had lost precious years with his kids and wife. He was now getting positive feedback from his family.

At all times, Robert and I talked choices, consequences, and applications. We talked of self-respect and respect for others as shown in communication techniques. Each session brought up new material from either 9/11, his past, or some reaction from his wife and kids. I talked with Robert's wife three times and suggested that they might consider marital counseling as a means by which to begin working together.

We evaluated our goals and set some new ones. Robert wanted to try marital counseling because he had begun to see that his wife wasn't all to blame; no, like himself, she had some issues they could tackle together. He still felt a bit insecure and wanted to prevent the return of his nightmares as well as those behaviors that had alienated his wife and children. This signaled the beginning of the last stage.

Some clients leave therapy at this stage because they feel better and stronger. There are other reasons for this. One may be an insurance limit on sessions. Some insurance companies have forms the client fills out regarding his or her progress. If there is good progress, the insurance company may not approve further sessions. Often these companies will reinstate the sessions if a relapse occurs. For this reason I don't fight the decisions unless the client is still not functioning well. I have had mostly good cooperation from insurance case managers. However, occasionally they do need further proof that more sessions are in order.

It is imperative to encourage the client to stay in therapy long enough to have a plan for relapses. These are likely, because therapy is the process of breaking old harmful patterns that once protected us from pain. This is not easy. I encourage clients to take notes in session, and about one third do. They then have reminders of what to practice between sessions and after termination of therapy. This helps solidify the client's inner strength and self-control.

We finally spread out three sessions over two months to end the treatment. In each session, I asked Robert what skills had been gained, what fears might have surfaced, how they were handled, and how this might be improved. I also explored what new beliefs have been gained, what learning and techniques have been acquired in order to become re-energized, and how the future needs to be envisioned.

If difficulties occur, I encourage clients to give me a call or call the insurance company and set up a session. I have had clients return after a lapse of months or years. They may have a new situation or trauma they need to assess and want guidance rather than therapy. In the meantime, many of them have practiced who they are, are living life on their own terms, and are working problems out with loved ones. This was the case with Robert.

Treatment for Children

Though there are some similarities in the therapy process used to treat adults and the one used for children—both processes involve such things as compassion, helping with connections, coping with symptoms, providing options, and proposing new skills—there are distinct differences in certain techniques. The timing, forms of expression, ways of talking, and material presented must be tailored to the individual, taking into consideration age, maturity, background, and severity of symptoms. The following case will give but one brief example of the many strategies that a therapist can use with children.

Becky's mother called me after Becky began having nightmares and panic attacks related to 9/11. Becky, nine years old, saw the repeated broadcasts on television of collapsing towers and discussions about terrorists and terrorism. Her parents talked animatedly about the events and this filled the family environment with anxiety. Mom and Dad tried to comfort Becky and allay her fears by pointing out that the attacks were over and she would be safe within her own surroundings. However, the nightmares didn't stop. There was no escape from 9/11 for Becky, due to repeated TV coverage, playground talk, new school security measures, and because she and her family were even searched at a familiar entertainment park.

Many of the strategies for dealing with Type A Night Terrors, which are listed in chapter 5, are applicable to recurring nightmares in children. I recommended that Becky's parents keep a log and asked her some of the same questions that appear in the "Notes and Log" section of that chapter. The most pertinent to nightmares are: when did they begin, how frequent, how severe, how many episodes per month, and was there screaming, crying, or talking? It is also important to note the time of occurrence, whether the child napped during the day, what stresses and interpersonal problems are in the child's life, and whether or not the child continually ingests caffeine or sugar before bedtime. This needs to be done before bringing the child to therapy.

One advantage in treating single-incident trauma-related nightmares as opposed to Type A Night Terrors is that there is no mystery about what caused the fear. Neither Becky's parents nor I had to spend time determining the cause of her discomfort. It was clear that she had been traumatized because of 9/11. We didn't have to guess whether her symptoms were the result of common daily fears of childhood. However, we did need to determine if she had suffered child abuse or chronic traumas in the past. But again, those parents who come forward in a timely manner and openly seek help are usually the ones with genuine, loving regard for their children.

At the initial session I asked Becky's mother to come into the office without her in order to tell me about their family and their response to 9/11. It became clear that the parents had done a good job of parenting and were genuinely concerned. I checked for child abuse by using the intake history previously described. The mother had already filled out a preliminary log. Children are usually more free and open when parents are not in the room. So, I explained to Becky's mother that the therapy would be more effective if during our earlier sessions she would stay in the waiting room. She agreed. Although this is preferable, it may not always be possible with very young children, especially if their trust of people has been severely shaken by trauma or abuse. I also explained that I would need to talk with Becky's parents as therapy progressed, either by phone or in separate sessions as needed. I usually set up weekly or biweekly sessions with the child during the earlier stages of therapy.

When Becky's mother finally brought her into my office for the first session alone with me, I asked the child if it would be okay for her mother to wait in the outer room. Becky agreed. During the session I began by engaging Becky in friendly, lighthearted conversation in order to put her at ease and develop a rapport with her. I acquainted the child with the playroom in my office and asked her what she would like to do first. She said she wanted to draw. I asked her to draw a picture of something she likes. We had a large selection of crayons and drawing paper. She drew a picture of her family and we talked about it. It was clear from the drawing that she had a supportive family. Then I asked her about what bothered her. She brought up how scary 9/11 was. We left discussion of that real situation until a later session when she might be more ready to confront the reality of it.

In the next session we returned to how scary 9/11 was, but I directed the discussion away from the real situation by asking Becky if she had any dreams or nightmares. When she said yes, I asked her to draw them. She used a black crayon to draw a ghost-like figure in the center of the page. The figure had red eyes and a hand sticking out. Its finger was pointing at a girl in the corner with a green dress and a sad face. When I asked her about the picture, she said that this nightmare came to her "a lot" and that she was afraid to sleep. I asked her what the figures meant to her, what happened in the nightmare, what her feelings were at the time, and whether she had ever experienced similar feelings before. This brought us back to 9/11. I again directed the conversation away from the real situation.

Instead, we talked about what she usually did when she was afraid at night and what she might do about it next time. As we brainstormed, she suddenly smiled and said she could have a flashlight under her pillow. She embellished the idea by saying, "If I wake up, I can shine it around the room and see that no one is there." I asked her how she thought she would feel about trying her flashlight idea. "Then I could feel safe," Becky replied. I continued by asking her what she might do if she still felt a little frightened. "I can go get Dad," was her reply. She had been in the habit of going to her parents' room and sleeping with them whenever she awakened from a nightmare. Wanting her to leave with something definite to do about her situation, I then asked if she would be willing to try the flashlight plan the next time she got scared at night. She assured me she would, and while still in my office, she explained to her mother what she planned to do.

When they came in for the third session, I asked Becky how the flashlight idea worked. She replied that there were no nightmares for the first two nights, but that on the third night the nightmares returned and seemed scarier than ever. On that night, she again ran for Dad and ended up sleeping with her parents. The next night Mom and Dad encouraged her to try the flashlight again. The nightmare returned, but Dad suggested they go back to her room and use the flashlight together in order to see that there was no danger. This procedure made it possible for Becky to go to sleep successfully again in her own room for the next few days. Although it was again unsuccessful on the night before she came back to my office, the flashlight procedure had already demonstrated the importance of trying new ways to solve problems as a means of finding new skills.

At the fourth session I asked Becky to draw the nightmare again. I noticed that the black figure was smaller and a little to the left of center. It still had red eyes and was pointing at the girl, whom she had drawn somewhat larger. She said the nightmare was still scary. This time I asked her what being scary was about, and what she was afraid of. She said that the figure ran after her and made her wake up screaming. We talked about whether dreams had power, whether the people in the dream were real, and whether they were like moving pictures. Becky picked up her picture and moved it back and forth. "You mean like this?" she asked. "Could it be possible, do you think?" I replied. Then I asked her to redraw the nightmare again and this time to make it the way she would like it to be. She drew the menacing figure in black, made the eyes a bright yellow, and made the girl not only bigger but also with a flashlight in her hand. I asked her if she wanted to continue using the flashlight to be sure her bedroom was safe. She promised that she would.

The foundation of therapy is to provide a comfortable, non-threatening environment in the hopes of facilitating some connections. As already explained in chapter 5, dreaming has a purpose similar to that of therapy, in that it is also trying to make emotional and behavioral connections. The next step is using this new awareness to learn skills for handling life's challenges.

In the second stage of therapy the child can reach beyond the trauma. The symptoms have begun to lessen and the child can contemplate the real events. At each session I ask the parent(s) to tell me what they have done to support the child and if they see relapse and/or progress. I ask them if they have any concerns. As often as possible I ask the child to share with the parent what he or she needs. Teaching the child in session how to speak of his or her needs is important to recovery. During this process we talk about the child's many different feelings and laugh a lot as we practice situations and responses while discussing the feelings that they evoke.

By the next session, Becky and I were able to talk about 9/11, not in terms of nightmares, but in terms of the real situation. I now could build upon her strengths by asking what frightening situations she had been in, such as while walking to school, while on the playground, or while watching scary movies. What has she said to herself in such situations? How has she handled getting help? How did it work out? At the same time, each session continued to deal with the nightmares, if they happened to return, and with what she would do if other nightmares happened to come along. We even imagined some nightmares that were funny and frightening at the same time.

There are also other tools that we have developed for use when relapses occur. The child might want to have a conversation with puppets or try to exchange good images for bad ones in nightmares, or reenact a situation in a sandtray.

The positive accomplishments of my sessions with Becky thus far acted as a signal to me that we were now ready to begin the final stage of therapy. In that stage I usually ask children for permission to bring their parents into the session. I also ask them if there are any fears they may still have and want to talk about. If so, we address those fears. Then I ask if they will share any pictures, ideas, and activities that they believe will help with future times of fear. This provides me with an opportunity to see the interaction of the family, even though I have given and gotten feedback from the parents separately during past sessions. By this time, I usually ask to see the child only every two weeks, then every three weeks. I also make it clear that if a problem comes up afterwards, the parents should give me a call.

The object of Becky's sessions was the deepening of self-control, self-confidence, and willingness to learn and to reach out to resources. Although it's much too early to gauge the long-term effectiveness of her treatment, much of what we tried did work to diminish her nightmare problem. At the time of this writing, a point had been reached where all involved were confident that a serious relapse was unlikely.

Readers wishing to acquire some deeper understandings of the different manifestations of trauma and anxiety in children of all ages might read *The Emotional Problems of Normal Children* by Stanley Turecki, M.D., with Sarah Wernick, Ph. D., *Monsters Under the Bed and Other Childhood Fears* by Steven W. Gerber, Ph. D., and Mary Anne Daniels Gerber, Ph. D., and *Your Anxious Child: How Parents and Teachers Can Relieve Anxiety in Children* by John Dacey and Lisa Fiore. As parents we can all use help formulating new techniques for helping children develop character and overcome trauma.

Concluding Thoughts

All severe trauma not only weakens self-confidence, self-esteem, and well-being; it often shakes or destroys the spiritual beliefs of its victims as well. This can become a major roadblock to recovery from nightmares or night terrors. Study after study has shown that those who have faith in some kind of spiritual force greater than themselves have a better chance of gaining and maintaining physical, mental, and emotional health.

Traumatic experiences often cause victims to question the ultimate fairness, if not the actual existence of a creator. "If there is a creator, then why was this tragedy allowed to happen?" is a phrase commonly heard in the aftermath of traumatic events. While searching for a helpful answer to that crucial question, some sufferers might be soothed by the belief that everything is controlled by the Creator for some higher purpose. Others are helped by the belief that the Creator gave all mankind free will and does not interfere. Acquiring belief in a higher Spiritual Force is one of the ways that victims of severe trauma can develop a better understanding and ultimate acceptance of the fact that tragedy is an unfortunate though widespread and unavoidable part of reality. Based on realizations such as these, trauma victims can be encouraged to work toward the restoration of their faith in a previously held set of positive spiritual beliefs or toward the acquisition of new ones.

Another consequence of severe trauma is a loss of trust in other people, which can cause victims to develop an exaggerated fear of being hurt again. This is often marked by emotional as well as physical withdrawal from the world. While severe traumas can cause us to suppress even our most healthy vulnerabilities, restoring an individual's willingness to take reasonable risks is essential in order for long-term healing to take place.

We are all relational beings who need to interact positively with other people in order to achieve emotional stability and balance in our lives. It is our human vulnerabilities that help us to make these valuable connections with others. Victims need to realize that by retreating into themselves and thereby temporarily numbing the pain, they will neither improve their emotional well-being nor strengthen their ability to defend themselves from harm. Recovery is not a journey to do in isolation. When reaching out and joining together with others, including other survivors of trauma, victims have a better chance of full recovery.

Once we have embraced our vulnerability and survived our pain, we can begin to relate to others and ourselves. Fear and pain provide us an opportunity to learn, to grow, and to bond. This moves us beyond our defenses against fear and into hope. All trauma-related symptoms remind us to closely examine our past and present. However, night terrors and nightmares specifically signal the need for correct diagnosis, meaningful connections, and truly effective solutions. The horror of personal and/or national trauma demands that we rise above complacency, recognize our strengths and weaknesses, and reevaluate our beliefs, values, and priorities. We need to become open to information, introspection, dialogue, and change in order to achieve emotional health and sound, stress-free sleep.

References

1. Dement W: *The Promise of Sleep*. New York: Delacorte, 1999.

2. Peck M Scott: *People of the Lie*. New York: Simon and Schuster, 1983.

3. *Diagnostic and Statistical Manual of Mental Disorders—Fourth Edition* (DSM-IV). Washington, DC: American Psychiatric Association, 1994.

4. Nemeroff C, Miller A, Bonsall R, Wilcox M, Graham Y, Heit S, Newport D, Heim C: "Pituitary-adrenal and autonomic responses to stress in women after sexual and physical abuse in childhood." *Journal of the American Medical Association* 2000; 284, 5.

5. Knapp S: "The nightmare, psychological and biological foundations." In *Night Terrors in Children and Adults: Emotional and Biological Factors*, edited by H. Kellerman. New York: Columbia University Press, 1987.

6. Dotto L: *Losing Sleep*. New York, William Morrow, 1990.

7. Webb W: *Sleep*. Massachusetts, Anker Publishing, 1992.

8. Marshall J: "The treatment of night terrors associated with the posttraumatic syndrome." *American Journal of Psychiatry* (March 1975); 132:3.

9. Eitinger L, Schwarz D: *Strangers in the World.* Vienna: Hans Huber Publishers, 1981.

10. Glod C, Teicher M, Hartman C, Harakal T: "Increased nocturnal activity and impaired sleep maintenance in abused children." *Journal of American Child and Adolescent Psychiatry* (September 1997); 36:9.

11. Eitinger L: *Concentration Camp Survivors in Norway and Israel.* The Hague: Martinus Nijhoff, 1972.

12. Eitinger L: "Anatomy of the Auschwitz death camp." In *Auschwitz—A Psychological Perspective,* edited by Y Gutman, M Berenbaum. Washington, DC: U.S. Holocaust Memorial Museum, 1994.

13. Kales J, Kales A, Soldatos CR, Caldwell AB, Charney DS, Martin ED: "Night terrors, clinical characteristics and personality patterns." *Archives of General Psychiatry* (1980); 37:1413–1417.

14. Fisher C, Kahn E, Edwards A, Davis DM: "A psychophysiological study of nightmares and night terrors." *Journal of Nervous and Mental Disease* (1973); 157:2.

15. Chodoff P: "Late effects of the concentration camp syndrome." *Archives of General Psychiatry* (1962); 7:323–333.

16. Leopold R, Dillon H: "Psycho-anatomy of a disaster." American Journal of Psychiatry (1963); 119:913–921.

17. Neylan T, Marmar C, Metzler T, Weiss D, Zatzick D, Delucchi K, Wu R, Schoenfeld F: "Sleep disturbances in the Vietnam generation." *American Journal of Psychiatry* (1998); 155:7.

18. Terr L: "Children of Chowchilla, a study of psychic trauma." *Psychoanalytic Study of the Child* (1979); 34:547–624.

19. Kales A, Soldatos CR, Bixler EO, Ladda, RL, Charney, DS, Weber, G, Schweitzer, PK: "Heredity factors in sleepwalking and night terrors." *British Journal of Psychiatry* (1980); 137:111–118.

20. Carlson C, White D: "Night terrors: a clinical and empirical review." *Clinical Psychology Review* (1982); 2:455–467.

21. Robinson S, Rapaport J, Durst R, Rapaport M, Rosca P,

Metzer S, Zilberman L: "The late effects of Nazi persecution among elderly Holocaust survivors." *Acta Psychiatrica Scandinavica* (1991); 82:311–314.

22. Schmolling P: "Human reactions to the Nazi concentration camps: a summing up." *Journal of Human Stress* (1984); 10:108–120.

23. Rosen J, Reynolds CF III, Yeager AL, Houck PR, Hurwitz, LF: "Sleep disturbances in survivors of the Nazi Holocaust." *American Journal of Psychiatry* (1991); 148:62–66.

24. Rogers A, Wingert P, Hayden T: "Why the young kill" (Special Issue). *Newsweek* (May 3, 1999); 133:32–35.

25. Garland E, Smith D: "Simultaneous prepubertal onset of panic disorder, night terrors, and somnambulism." *Journal of the American Academy of Child and Adolescent Psychiatry* (1991); 30:4.

26. Kales J, Kales A, Soldatos CR, Chamberlin K, Martin ED: "Sleepwalking and night terrors related to febrile illness." *American Journal of Psychiatry* (1979); 136:9.

27. Hartmann E: *Dreams and Nightmares*. New York: Plenum Trade, 1998.

28. Terr L: "Psychic trauma in children." *American Journal of Psychiatry* (1981); 138:1.

29. Mahowald MW, Rosen GW: "Parasomnias in children." *Pediatrician* (1990); 17:21–31.

30. Kales J, Cadieux R, Soldatos CR, Kales A: "Psychotherapy with night terror patients." *American Journal of Psychotherapy* (1982); XXXVI-3.

31. Hartmann E: Two case reports: "Night terrors with sleepwalking—a potentially lethal disorder." *Journal of Nervous and Mental Disease* (1983); 171:8.

32. Bettelheim B: "Individual and mass behavior in extreme situations." *Journal of Abnormal Social Psychology* (1943); 38:417–452.

33. Eitinger L: "Coping with aggression." *Mental Health Society* (1974); 1297–301.

34. Chu J: *Rebuilding Shattered Lives*. New York: John Wiley & Sons, 1998.

35. Santrock, JW: *Life-Span Development* (7th edition). New York: McGraw-Hill College, 1999.

36. Morrissette P: "Post-traumatic stress disorder in childhood sexual abuse." *Child and Adolescent Work Journal* (1999); 16:2.

37. Eitinger L: "Essential papers on posttraumatic stress disorder." In *Organic and Psychosomatic Aftereffects of Concentration Camp Imprisonment*, edited by M. Horowitz. New York: New York University Press, 1999.

38. Magid K, McKelvy C: *High Risk Children Without a Conscience*. New York: Bantam Books, 1989.

39. Fisher C, Kahn E, Edwards A, Davis DM, Fine J: "A psychophysiological study of nightmares and night terrors." *Journal of Nervous and Mental Disease* (1974); 158:3.

40. Riley T, editor: *Clinical Aspects of Sleep and Sleep Disturbance*. Boston: Butterworth-Heinemann, 1985.

41. DeAngelis B: *Are You the One for Me*. New York: Dell Publishing, 1992.

42. Schlessinger L: *Ten Stupid Things Men Do To Mess Up Their Lives*. New York: Cliff Street Books, 1997.

43. Fenig S, Levav I: "Demoralization and social supports among Holocaust survivors." *Journal of Nervous and Mental Disease* (1991); 179:3.

44. Brownlee S: "Mother love betrayed." *U.S. News & World Report* (1996); vol. 120, no. 17: 59.

45. Begley S: "The nursery's littlest victims." *Newsweek* (1997); vol. 130, no. 12: 72.

46. Godfrey K: "The disease of deceit." *Nursing Times* (1998); vol. 94, no. 30: 24.

47. Southall D: "Covert video recordings of life-threatening child abuse." *Journal of the American Medical Association* (1998); vol. 279, no. 2: 9.

48. Donald T, Jureidini J, DeAngelis D: "Munchausen syn-

drome by proxy." *Archives of Pediatrics & Adolescent Medicine* (1996); vol. 150, no. 7: 757.

49. Souid A, Keith D, Cunningham A: "Munchausen syndrome by proxy." *Clinical Pediatrics* (1998); vol. 37, no. 8: 497.

50. Williams R, Karacan I, Moore C: *Sleep Terrors. Sleep Disorders, Diagnosis and Treatment.* New York: John Wiley & Sons, 1985.

51. Lillywhite A, Wilson S, Nutt D: "Successful treatment of night terrors and somnambulism with paroxetine." *British Journal of Psychiatry* (1994); 164.

52. Genevieve J, Berman L, Bryk M: "How her mother hurt her . . . in the name of love." *Redbook* (1998); vol. 190, no. 4: 91.

53. Carranza C: "Terror after dark." *Family Therapy News* (1999); vol. 30, no. 4.

54. *Orange County Register,* February 28, 2002.

55. Grant R: *The Way of the Wound.* Oakland, CA: Robert Grant, 1996.

56. Barrett D: *Trauma and Dreams.* Cambridge, MA: Harvard University Press, 1996.

57. Delaney G: *In Your Dreams.* San Francisco: Harper, 1997.

58. Miller A: *The Truth Will Set You Free.* New York: Basic Books, 2001.

59. Viscott D: *Emotional Resilience: Simple Truths for Dealing with the Unfinished Business of Your Past.* New York: Three Rivers Press, 1996.

60. Solomon J, Carol G: *Attachment Disorganization.* New York: Guilford Press, 1999.

61. Levine P, Frederick A: "The Feeling of What Happens: Body and Emotion in the Making of Consciousness." New York: Harcourt, 1999.

62. Parnell L: *EMDR in the Treatment of Adults Abused as Children.* New York: W.W. Norton, 1999.

63. Tannen D: *The Argument Culture: Stopping America's War Of Words.* New York: Ballantine, 1998.

64. Bradley B: "An intimate look into emotionally focused

therapy: an interview with Susan M. Johnson." *Marriage &*
Family: A Christian Journal (2001); vol. 4, no. 2.

65. Higgins G: *Resilient Adults: Overcoming a Cruel Past.*
San Francisco: Jossey-Bass Publishers, 1994.

66. *Orange County Register,* October 26, 2002.   •

67. *Orange County Register*, November 9, 2002.